BELLY BUSTIN' TIPS

You Can Use on ANY Diet

Nancy Lee McCaskill

and Michael Vernon

QUAILS' NEST PUBLISHING

MURRELLS INLET, SC

Copyright © 2015 Quails' Nest Publishing

All rights reserved.

ISBN-13: 978-0-9864005-2-0

DEDICATION

My interest in general nutrition began in 4-H at a very early age. But the people to whom I am dedicating this book are people who fostered my interest in the nutrition of weight loss. Without either of them, I'd never have been able to learn enough about nutrition to open my clinics nor would I ever have had the self-esteem to run a conglomerate of businesses on my own.

My aunt, Etha M. Bailey, not only shares a birthday with me, but also shares my passion for studying nutrition. She is a retired registered dietitian and initially provided the seed money for my first clinic, took me on many continuing ed courses with her, wrote and rewrote menus, helped with our cookbooks, and was available for countless questions for me and for clients. My friend, Beth Rodamer, has been like a second mother and was also my initial trainer, supporter, and mentor. She has always believed in me, well before I believed in myself. I will be forever grateful for all they did for me, but most of all for their love, their encouragement, and the huge belief they had in me. Both of these women have been the wind beneath my wings. Bless you, and I hope you continue to help others fly.

Written by the Mary Kay of Weight Loss

"Lee's two qualities that make this book so special is that she has a strong, relentless passion for helping people and for researching subjects she is interested in, like weight loss. Having known her for 30 years, I can tell you, Lee really cares that you succeed and wants to hear from you *personally*. Rest assured she put a lot of time and effort into the production of what you're about to read, and it *will* be phenomenal because that's just the way she rolls."
Bob Samara, President, Image Unlimited

Get Fit in the Gym to Lose Weight in the Kitchen

"Blending fun and science, Lee creates a recipe for success. She combines a simple, flexible, and tasty cuisine, as well as a host of tools to help you stay on track with healthy eating and tons of tips."

"Exercise is great, but your hard work in the gym can be wasted if you aren't working as hard in the kitchen. Once you understand how the two work together, like bank deposits and withdrawals, you can manage your fat account like you do your checkbook. This takes effort, practice and the willingness to invest in your success, just like reading this book."
Bonnie Pfiester, Max Fitness Club, Vero Beach, FL, BCx Trainer

Fix the emotional as well as physical part of your temporary weight problem for the permanent solution.

"The foundation to transformation is really a promise...a promise you keep to yourself on a consistent basis. Each promise kept—each brick laid—builds a strong foundation of self-esteem and confidence that is rock-solid and indestructible." That is what Michael Vernon does in his Life Choices section of this book. You can't have physical transformation without emotional transformation first.
Chris Powell, Transformation Specialist, Extreme Makeover

The Diet Doctors Rave About

"The Belly Buster Diet *IS* the diet doctors rave about: it helps improve a patient's cholesterol & blood pressure, as well as lose weight safely and effectively. Great for diabetics, people with IBS and hypothyroidism, too.
Dr. Joshua T. Watson, MD, gastroenterologist

CONTENTS

ACKNOWLEDGMENTS

We would like to express our gratitude to our editor Melissa Wuske and proofreader Jessica Resnick. Melissa's ability to play the devil's advocate and make a writer think what message they are conveying, to assemble like pieces of the pie together, and to rewrite when we got wordy or messy really helped mold this manuscript into something we could be proud of. Jennifer's attention to detail polished it and gave it the once over it needed. Both of them were professional and prompt, and we wish them much success in the future.

INTRODUCTION

Have you been on every diet on the planet and lost weight on each one, only to gain it back every time? Many of us have. This weight loss wobble is like being on a merry-go-round that you don't like and don't know how to dismount. When you finally do fall off, you are right back on the merry-go-round before you can say "celery sticks". No matter how hard you try, you are on that same merry-go-round again and again! If chronic repeat dieters knew what to do and why this happens, they would not be on diet after diet. If you relate to this, I have some Belly Bustin' Tips that will help you, no matter what diet you are currently following.

"I've been on diets all my life. I think I have lost over 875 pounds over my lifetime. I should be a charm on a charm bracelet, but I'm not." —Erma Bombeck

I was like you! I, too, have done enough weight loss plans to have my doctorate in dieting. I lost 40 pounds after the birth of my son over thirty years ago, only to gain it back and then revisit that merry-go-round more than a few times. Between my bouts with polycystic ovary syndrome (PCOS), thyroid disease, and mixed connective tissue disease (an autoimmune disorder), I kept packing on more and more weight. After peaking at my highest weight, I finally lost 90 pounds. But I was only able to do that because I'd learned to fix the yo-yo syndrome both physically and emotionally.

1) I studied how metabolism works to figure out how I could rev mine up. I was a microbiologist, for heaven's sake, with plenty of biology classes under my belt. (If I didn't know, I certainly don't expect you to know!)

2) I worked as hard on *me*, especially the emotional part of me, as I did dieting. I love the saying Oprah Winfrey shares frequently: "It's not what you're eating; it's what's eating you!" Until you fix the stressors and heal the pain, the weight stays. (I don't know too many people who are fat and who meditate and do yoga. Do you?)

A turning point in my perspective on my weight was when I saw an obese man at an auto dealership. He had the most beautiful car I had ever seen, with all the bells and whistles, and you could tell the guy had taken exquisite care of it. It was several years old, but it was as shiny as the day he bought it. The man was so heavy he could barely walk and was having trouble breathing. The clerk at the counter was fussing at him, "You know that body of yours—it is the only one you are ever going to get. If you would take as good of care of your body as you do that car…" A week later, I was back in the dealership and the man's car was for sale because he had died at age 48.

What if I gave you a car, any car you wanted, with one caveat: This is the only car you are ever going to have the rest of your life. How well would you take care of it? I am sure you would wash and wax it almost daily; you would change the oil frequently; you would put conditioner on the seats so the leather wouldn't crack; you would rub down the tires so they wouldn't dry rot. You would work on that car daily since it's the only one you'll ever get!

Well, guess what? You *are* only getting *one* body! How well do you take care of it? Are you taking exquisite care of it? Is it time for a 45,000-calorie checkup? Do you check your fluids regularly? Have you gotten rid of old spare tires? If not, this book will put you on the right track and help you rev up that engine.

The purpose of this book is to provide you with the understanding of how your metabolism works, as well as some tips you can use to reach your goal on any diet. It addresses the physical side (Section I) and the emotional or mental side (Section II) of losing weight. My son, gastroenterologist Major Joshua T. Watson, M.D., has helped me with the explanation of metabolism and the section on irritable bowel syndrome (IBS). Section II of the book is written by my friend and partner, Michael Vernon, based on the seven-class course, Life Choices, that he teaches in my clinics. He is a behavioral therapist who will teach you exercises that will help you stop sabotaging yourself. One of the themes of Michael's classes is a quote of his that I love: "*Every* choice you make in life helps determine your destiny tomorrow, including what you had for breakfast this morning."

After reading our tips, many of you will probably want to join us on our journey to **commit to be fit** (please join us at http://www.2bfitweek.wordpress.com), and I hope you do! Michael's Life Choices classes are available by teleconference, and our weight management system, the Belly Buster Diet, is available both locally on the Treasure Coast of Florida through Before and After Weight Loss Clinics and nationwide through our network of consultants, Belly Busters. To make an appointment locally, call 772-429-1110 or 772-562-3601 and ask for the "book special". To become a client of ours outside of the Treasure Coast area, please or visit our website, http://www.bestdietsource.com/ and click on the link on the right that says "health profile". A consultant will call you and use the medical history in your health profile to do a 30-minute metabolic assessment. It's kept completely confidential, just like in a doctor's office. Then we can tell you more about our program, go over any costs, and determine how long it would take get to your goal weight. Be as accurate as possible on your health profile, as this also tells us which herbal supplements and vitamins are right for you. If you prefer, simply call our toll-free number, 1-800-657-5402.

We offer six different nutritional plans and the consultant will go over the one best suited for your medical needs. Please do not share your menu with others, as men and women of different weights are on different caloric intakes, and people with certain health concerns are on different menus. The Belly Buster Diet is low-carb and low-fat. It is a rapid weight loss program, so one of our counselors will need to monitor your progress via phone and email to ensure your success as well as answer any questions. If you should have any unusual side effects, these counselors will know what to do to remedy them. Any doctor will tell you that you should not attempt to lose more than a pound a week on your own, so our counselors' professional services are vital to your

3

success. You can order our products via the website or on our toll-free line (1-888-657-5042). We carry protein supplements, herbal supplements, vitamins, Wisdom Natural Brands Sweet Leaf™ Stevia, Walden Farms™ products, and Tropical Spa Body Wraps™. Free shipping and biweekly product specials are available for out-of-town clients.

Disclaimer: We are *not* affiliated in *any* way with Before-N-After Weight Loss in California, even though their logo is similar to ours. Although Before and After Weight Loss Clinic has been our trademark since July 2000, they have insisted on using our name since 2007. We *do not* endorse their program, and it is not to be confused with ours.

SECTION I:
THE PHYSICAL SIDE
OF WEIGHT LOSS

Nancy Lee McCaskill & Michael Vernon

1 A DOZEN DIRTY DIET MYTHS

We have all heard the same recurring "rules" for dieting. Just like rumors, you never know who started them, and like gossip, some are just myths! So which information is correct? Get the diet dogma out of your head so you can move ahead. Here's the skinny on the top dozen myths I hear most often in my diet clinics.

Diet Myth #1: You shouldn't eat after 6 p.m.—the food turns right into fat.
Your weight is affected by your collective calories over the whole the day, whether you eat late or not. The truth is, you should eat about three hours before you retire for the night to allow time for digestion, but what time that is depends on what time you go to bed. If you go to bed at 9:00 p.m., it would be best not to eat after 6:00 p.m. If you are going to bed at midnight, it is fine to eat at 9:00 p.m. Just give your body time to digest your food, but try not to have more than a four- to five-hour stretch between meals and try to have one portion-controlled, healthy snack in-between.
   TIP: Try to eat fruits and heavy starches before 3:00 p.m. in order to burn them off when you are most active; however, you can have fruit later if you work out at night. Also, later in the day, eat low glycemic fruits rather than high glycemic ones (see chapter five "What Is the Glycemic Index?").

Diet Myth #2: Salads are always healthy; you can never go wrong with a salad.

Well, you can—salads can be loaded with calories and fat, depending on what toppings and dressing you choose. One ounce of shredded cheese has 10 grams of fat; avocado has 4.5 grams of fat per *small* slice; Caesar dressing has 22 grams of fat. If you add olives, buttered croutons, and dried fruit (all of which are high in both calories and carbohydrates), before you know it, you will gain weight while eating salad! The key to weight loss is to take in fewer calories than you burn. Too much of any one food, no matter how healthy, will sabotage your weight loss efforts. So, bottom line: Count the calories in a salad, even if you don't know anything else about it, like how many grams of fat or carbohydrates it has in it.

TIP: Knowledge is power! Invest in a carbohydrate and fat count book that lists the carbohydrate and fat content for various foods. Get familiar with which foods are primarily proteins, carbohydrates, and fats. For a quick, fun test of your knowledge on the basics, take the quiz at the end of this chapter.

Diet Myth #3: Diet soda is harmless, and you should drink it when you are dieting.

Researchers have discovered a link between obesity and artificial sweeteners used in diet soda. Purdue University conducted a study that found that rats fed artificial sweeteners before mealtime tended to eat more than rats fed sugar. In another study, they found that people who consumed three diet sodas per week were 40 percent more likely to be obese than people who did not consume diet sodas.

TIP: Pure water, rather than diet soda, is ideal when dieting because it helps flush melted fat as well as toxins out of your body. If you have a hard time making the transition from diet sodas to water, try using drops of flavored liquid Stevia in your water. Stevia is all-natural and will not interfere with your weight loss like carbonated drinks with sodium or artificially flavored drinks will. For your overall diet, limit your use of artificial sweeteners to no more than the equivalent of four packets per day and never use sweeteners that end in "–ol" (alcohol sugars). Also, Truvia® contains erythritol, an alcohol sugar that gives some people extreme bouts of gas, and it has 3 grams of carbohydrates per packet, and, in my opinion, is not a good choice for weight loss or for people with irritable bowel syndrome.

Diet Myth #4: Sea salt is a healthier version of regular salt.
Contrary to what you may have heard, the body cannot tell much difference between the two. Both contain roughly 2,300 milligrams of sodium per teaspoon. It is best to reduce sodium intake and increase potassium intake (with melons and vegetables, not higher carb bananas) when dieting. If you experience leg cramps, then try increasing your sodium intake, as you may have cut it too severely.

TIP: If you crave salt, try some of the Mrs. Dash and McCormick seasonings with no salt. I also use lots of fresh spices from www.SpiceHunter.com to cut down on the amount of sodium I consume. Consult a physician before using a salt substitute like No Salt; certain medications, like blood thinners, diuretics, ibuprofen, and aspirin, may have dangerous reactions with the potassium chloride in salt substitutes and may even lead to heart failure or sudden death.

Diet Myth #5: Certain foods, like cabbage soup or grapefruit, can burn fat.
It's true that these foods are low in calories, but there is no scientific basis that diets based on these foods will help you lose long-term weight. If you lose weight when you eat them, it is probably because you are substituting them for other higher calorie foods in your diet than you normally eat. Also, foods with more fiber in them may make you feel full faster and help take some of the carbs of other foods out of your body during digestion and elimination.

TIP: Use lipotropic (fat-burning) herbs to burn fat. Some of the more popular ones include garcinia cambogia, green coffee bean, guarana, inositol, African mango, and bitter melon. Be sure to buy from a health practitioner who knows the potential drug interactions of these products or consult your physician before taking products containing any herbal formulas.

Diet Myth #6: Fat-free foods are diet foods.
When food manufacturers remove the fat from food, they often add sugar—and therefore calories and carbs—to add back the flavor. Snackwell's™ do not make diet food! In fact, when people

are given foods marked as low-fat, they consume 25 to 44 percent more calories than when foods are not labeled that way and are, in essence, full-fat or contain that food's normal fat content, according to Brian Wansink, Ph.D., author of *Mindless Eating: Why We Eat More Than We Think* and director of Cornell University's Food and Brand Lab. They also underestimate the total number of calories they're consuming. According to Wansink, most snack foods are lower in calories by only about 11 percent compared to their full-fat versions, yet people typically believe that low-fat foods are 44 percent lower in calories. What's more, "They believe they are *entitled* to eat more because they sacrificed by eating a low-fat food," says Wansink.

TIP: Read labels. A fat-free food is almost always much higher in carbohydrates than its higher-fat substitute. Sometimes neither will be right for your diet plan. Check for carb, fat, and sodium content.

Diet Myth #7: Vodka has fewer calories than other types of alcohol, so it is better for you while dieting.

First of all, an ounce of hard liquor (gin, vodka, rum, whiskey, or scotch) contains 64 calories for 80 proof varieties and 80 calories for those that are 100 proof. None is better than another. The problem is that most people don't have just one ounce per drink, nor do they usually have just one drink. The calorie-laden mixers, such as orange juice and soda, can add 500 more calories to your libations.

TIP: See chapter nine, "Handling Holidays," for tips on booze while you lose.

Diet Myth #8: If you skip one meal a day, like breakfast, you can lose weight faster.

This may work temporarily, but it will eventually backfire on you, just like 500-calorie diets and diets that replace a meal with a cookie or shake do. When people skip meals or decrease their calories significantly (to fewer than 1,000 calories per day), they actually decrease their metabolism. Their bodies go into starvation mode and try to store fat to conserve energy. The metabolic rate can actually decrease as much as 10 to 15 percent, and your body will hold on to fat and burn lean muscle instead.

TIP: *Always* eat three meals a day. Keep high protein nutritional bars on hand in case you are in a situation where you cannot eat a full meal. If you have trouble remembering to eat, set an alarm on your cell phone to go off every four or five hours to remind you. If you snack between meals, it should be protein; if you are diabetic, the between-meal snacks should be a fruit with a protein.

Diet Myth #9: If you are exercising and sticking to your diet and still haven't lost this month, you must be gaining muscle tissue.
It takes more than a month and quite a lot of exercise to build up any significant muscle tissue. Most people who say this are in absolute denial that they are cheating or whether they have exercised long enough for muscle tissue to have developed.

TIP: Always keep a food journal, and show it to someone to whom you can be accountable. If you are on a low-carb diet, use ketone sticks at least once per week to monitor yourself. The sticks pick up the ketones given off in your urine when you are in ketosis to show that you are burning fat. Ketone sticks are available on our website for less than you can get them in your local pharmacy.

Diet Myth #10: Bananas are the best source of potassium while dieting.
Doctors often tell you to eat bananas for potassium when your levels are low, and that is fine—unless you are trying to lose weight. While bananas are often touted as an excellent source of potassium to prevent leg cramps, they are also very high in carbohydrates. One-half of a medium banana (about 7 inches) has 24 grams of carbohydrates. Many fruits have half the carbohydrates that bananas do, and dieters can choose other foods that have similar amounts of potassium with fewer calories. Here is a list of lower carb foods with high potassium content: watermelon, broccoli, spinach, cantaloupe, yogurt, papaya, salmon, mushrooms, and strawberries. While maintaining your weight after the diet phase, apricots and sun-dried tomatoes are both excellent sources of potassium, but they are slightly higher in carbohydrates. Most clinical-grade protein supplements also have added potassium.

There are three reasons why you may need more potassium while dieting:

1) The increase in drinking water may flush out some of your potassium.

2) The increase in exercise may warrant more potassium lost from perspiration.

3) The dietary restrictions of your menus may not be providing enough potassium if you are making your own choices rather than having a dietitian or nutritionist choosing foods for you.

One way you will know you need to increase your potassium intake is muscle cramps, particularly in the legs. If you have cramps, add the fruits and vegetables listed above back to your diet for a few days; and if you are on a diet plan that incorporates protein supplements, choose the ones with the most potassium in them for a few days. However, the cramps may be due to low sodium rather than low potassium, since drinking a lot of water may flush out other electrolytes besides just potassium. If you are already eating these foods high in potassium, then try adding a pinch more salt to your diet each day before worrying about adding more potassium.

TIP: Listen to your nutritionist or dietitian for your nutritional issues and your doctor for medical issues. Nutrition professionals do not have medical courses in college, and medical doctors usually do not have nutritional courses in medical school. If you get conflicting information, do not be afraid to say something. For instance, if you say to your doctor, "Bananas are not on my weight loss plan," a physician may instead prescribe you a prescription strength dose of potassium to take for a few days if he or she does not think you will get enough in other high-potassium foods you can eat.

Diet Myth #11: Egg yolks raise your cholesterol.

Eggs have gotten a bad rap because of the long-held belief that they raise cholesterol. While eggs raise dietary cholesterol (the amount you take in), this form of cholesterol, in contrast with blood serum cholesterol (the amount your body makes and retains), has not been significantly linked to heart disease. Eggs are a good source of protein for any meal and for snacking. Go ahead—eat the yolk! If you have high cholesterol, you can limit them to no more than two or three per day. They will actually help keep your insulin in check. If you use egg substitutes, use the ones with just egg whites and no unnatural ingredients. Eggs are great for making diet cheesecakes, soufflés, frittatas, omelets, and casseroles, all of which you can eat on the Belly Buster Diet. If you are on a different nutritional plan, check to see how many eggs you can have.

TIP: Keep boiled eggs in the refrigerator for quick snacks. Since they are high in protein and have only 70 calories, you won't blow your diet eating just one, and you will feel more satiated at meals. If you make deviled eggs, use only a small amount of mayonnaise and add mustard or Walden Farms fat-free dressings to it to give them more volume. (Walden Farms Thousand Island makes egg salad taste like it has pickles in it.)

Diet Myth #12: Juice fasting is a great way to slim down and cleanse.

Your kidneys, liver, and bladder do the job of cleansing quite nicely. Juices are high in sugar and can create chaos by sending blood sugar levels up then down, leaving you quite hungry. Even a lower-sugar juice is void of protein, a macronutrient that's crucial during weight loss to prevent loss of lean muscle mass, stabilize blood sugar, and rev up metabolism. Most registered dietitians say, "No, no, no!" to juice fasts. And, so will I!

TIP: Do not use commercial colon cleansers as an alternative way to cleanse, either. Overuse of those products strip your colon of the little hairs, called cilia, that pick up vital nutrients. The best alternative is to cleanse by eating foods with a lot of fiber. For one to two weeks eat lots of salads, and add a fruit and a vegetable at every meal in addition to whatever protein you are eating—except breakfast, where you can do a fruit and a high-fiber, sugar-free cereal or a starch with a calcium source, like yogurt, cheese, or some form of low-fat milk (soy, almond, or dairy). On the Belly Buster Diet, everyone starts with a detoxifying cleanse like this.

NOTES:_____

_____

_____

_____

_____

_____

_____

_____

_____

_____

_____

_____

_____

_____

What other myths have you heard that later proved to be untrue?_____

_____

_____

_____

_____

_____

2 WHAT IS METABOLISM?

"Metabolism" is the word used to describe how your body changes food into energy for all of your bodily processes. The word literally means "transformation". Both diet and exercise play important roles in regulating your body's metabolism. A healthy diet can help you lose weight and maintain a leaner body mass, while a regular exercise routine can tone your body and improve your general health. Your body's metabolism is running all the time—while you are exercising, while you are eating, and even while you are sleeping—to help your body do all of these things and more:

- create new cells and tissue
- maintain its temperature
- repair injuries
- perform all bodily activities

Metabolism is generally measured according to your basal metabolic rate (BMR). This is a calculation of how quickly your metabolism works when you are resting. Any health professional can calculate your BMR using special equipment. Your primary doctor or an endocrinologist can also do thyroid tests to determine how well your metabolism is working based on thyroid function. Those tests are not always reliable, but in this book, you will find a few tests you can take on your own to determine how well your metabolism is actually working.

So, how does your metabolism work? Metabolism is the rate at which your body burns calories from the food that you eat. Your body gets all of its energy from plant and animal products that you ingest daily, which we measure in calories. Your body breaks down what you eat into energy that it can use to run different cellular processes. Enzymes released by your pancreas and thyroid gland help to break your food down into sugars, amino acids, and fatty acids. These three types of energy are then absorbed into your bloodstream and transported to different cells in your body to help to run all of your body's different processes. Any excess energy is then stored as muscle or fat so that it can be used in the future.

Since metabolism is a rate of use, it is not always constant. When you sleep, it is slower than when you are exercising. Overall, your metabolism is higher when you exercise regularly. Just exercising three times a week for twenty minutes is enough to raise your metabolism! You can walk at a fast pace, outdoors or on a treadmill, ride a bike, or swim, and that is enough to keep it up.

TIP: Some dieters fail at dieting simply because they are exercising more than the protocol for their plan. As a result, they do not get enough calories to sustain the extra exercise and are always hungry and give up. If you insist on doing more exercise than your plan calls for, discuss it with your counselor to adjust your caloric intake so that you will have enough food to sustain you for your workouts. Once you reach maintenance goal weight and have a larger caloric intake, increase your exercise adding weight-bearing exercises and aerobic exercise, and alternate intensities to get more effective metabolic increases.

Many different factors affect metabolism. The most important factor is the amount of lean muscle mass that your body contains. Lean muscle mass burns energy all the time, even when you are not actively working out. It also burns more calories than any other part of your body. The more lean muscle mass you have, the higher your metabolism will be. Makes you want to exercise, doesn't it?

Your age, genetics, hormones, and body composition determine the rate of your metabolism. Age and genetics cannot be changed, but your hormones and body composition can be manipulated to a degree through exercise, the food you eat, the supplements you take, and how well you treat your body (like getting enough sleep, etc.).

So, let's look at these factors affecting metabolism:

- **Age:** As you age, your metabolism naturally slows down. This is, in part, because the body loses lean muscle mass over the years. Expect your metabolism to decline by about 2 percent every decade after the age of 20.

  TIP: By menopause or age 58, you should cut your caloric intake by one-third and increase your weight-bearing exercises.

- **Sex:** Men have naturally higher levels of lean muscle mass. This means that women will generally have lower metabolisms than men because muscle uses up to 90 percent more calories than any other tissue in your body. The more muscle you have, the more calories you will burn in a day. In addition to muscle mass, many other things like hormones, cortisol levels, water fluctuations, and chocolate cravings (imagine that!) can all hold women back from losing weight in ways that men don't experience.

  TIP: A woman can increase her metabolism during a diet by simply adding a protein supplement like the ones we have on the Belly Buster Diet. Protein provides the building blocks for muscle. You need about .4 to .5 grams of protein per pound of body weight. A woman weighing 160 pounds needs about 64 to 80 grams of protein daily. (Our protein comes in packets with 12 to 15 grams of protein and in flavored fruit drinks, gelatins, soups, and puddings—see our website, www.bestdietsource.com, for details.) Of course men can use a protein supplement, too, but don't make any bets with your partner on who will lose weight faster—he still has the edge!

  TIP: In addition to exercising and using protein supplements, another way to build muscle tissue is to use an inexpensive mineral supplement called chromium picolinate. A nice bonus of this wonder mineral is that, for most people, it helps you crave chocolate less and stabilizes your blood sugar, making dieting easier. This is especially good news for women during ovulation and in preparation for menses, when the body uses a lot of chromium and craves chromium-rich snacks like chocolate.

- **Height:** People who are taller have a greater surface area for their bodies to fuel. As result, taller people tend to have a more active metabolism and require more calories to stay energized. (I wish there was a tip for getting taller; I'd be the first to use it!)

- **Family history:** Your genetic makeup also plays a role. Some families have a naturally high metabolism, while others have a naturally low metabolism. Scientists have now discovered a gene that predisposes some families to be overweight, and they have found that a hormone called leptin is produced in different levels in different people. Leptin tells your brain how satiated you are. If your levels are high, you are not as satiated.

  TIP: Use a good quality raspberry ketone supplement to feel fuller faster and green coffee bean extracts to help change your metabolism. According to Dr. Sarah G. Kahn, raspberry ketone supplements work in two ways: 1) It increases your metabolism by increasing the release of a hormone called norepinephrine. This suppresses your appetite as it speeds up the metabolism; 2) Raspberry ketones also help your body make a protein-related hormone known as adiponectin that greatly lowers glucose levels. Green coffee bean extract is made from unroasted coffee beans. It is low in caffeine and high in chlorogenic acid. It has two main weight loss properties: it stimulates metabolism, literally changing it, and it instructs the body to start converting fat reserves into energy, which also helps lower glucose and insulin levels. We have both raspberry ketone supplements and green coffee bean extracts on our website, www.bestdietsource.com, and you can read more about them there.

- **Eating habits:** Food is fuel, or energy, for your body. The more often you eat, the more active and well fueled your metabolism will be. If you skip a meal, your body will enter starvation mode, and your metabolism will slow down to conserve energy for your brain and other organs. Any excess energy is stored as fat. Eat too much and it is stored as fat; eat too little and the storage is conserved.

  TIP: Never, ever participate in a weight loss program with less than 1,200 calories on its main menus, no matter what kind of "science" they tell you is behind it or what "doctor" they claim touted it. A perfect example of how the public can be deceived is the hCG diet, a diet on which a person eats only 500 calories while taking injections of urine from a pregnant horse. Despite the fact that it was deemed an ineffective diet in 1962 by the *Journal of the American Medical Association* and again in 1976 by the Federal Trade Commission (FTC), Kevin Trudeau made it massively popular in 2007 with the release of his book *The Weight Loss Cure "They" Don't Want You to Know About.* This infomercial fraudster was convicted in March 2014 after the FTC filed several actions against him for misrepresenting information in the book, including how effective hCG is. Unfortunately, dieters flocked to find the "cure" after his book came out, and hCG is still selling like crazy in weight loss clinics across the nation that are unethical enough to carry it. I don't care what kind of shot or cookie or lollipop someone gives you, if they starve you with only 500 calories to lose weight, it wasn't the high-priced sucker that made you lose the weight; it was the starvation diet—and in no way, shape, or form is that healthy! You have to eat to lose to keep it off *permanently* and not screw up your metabolism.

- **Exercise and metabolism:** Exercise also plays a key role in determining the rate at which your metabolism works. Exercise helps to increase metabolism in two ways:

    1) When you perform an activity, your metabolism will naturally speed up in order to burn up enough energy to fuel your bodily movements. Your metabolism will remain elevated for up to 12 hours after you exercise. **TIP:** Just 20 to 30 minutes of exercise, especially in the morning or midday, can make a tremendous difference in your weight loss efforts. Is it worth an extra pound per week, or even more, to get up 30 minutes earlier each morning or take half of your lunch hour to exercise?

    2) Exercise is a natural way to increase your metabolism because muscle burns more calories than fat. This is particularly true of strength training exercises, such as weight lifting and resistance exercises.

You have to take in 3,500 calories to make one pound; but if you walk around the block a couple of times, you only burn about 100 calories. Hardly seems fair, does it? The truth is that it is going to take a lot more effort on your nutritional planning than it is on your exercise plan, although both are a key to long-term success. A short time on a diet or a few months a year at the gym isn't going to cut it. Weight management is a *lifelong commitment* to eating healthy.

TIP: Whatever diet you choose, *always* participate in its maintenance program. Maintenance is always a different nutritional plan than the dieting plan, and it will teach you skills for keeping the weight off that you did not learn during the other phases of the diet. If psychological counseling is offered with your program, participate! If not, seek it on your own because food is an addiction, and a weight problem should be treated as such, even when metabolic problems are present.

Metabolic Problems
How well the organs that break down your food are functioning can affect your metabolism. Metabolic problems can be present at birth or can develop over time. Two of the organs we mentioned previously, the thyroid and pancreas, can cause two of the most common metabolic disorders if untreated.

- **Diabetes:** This condition is caused by an inappropriate response to your body's blood glucose (energy) levels. Diabetes is the result of a deficiency of insulin. In the case of Type 1, the body doesn't make enough insulin; with Type 2, the pancreas makes insulin, but the body is resistant to using it effectively. When you have diabetes and insulin levels are not normal, your body has trouble metabolizing the food you eat into energy. Diabetes can result in rapid weight loss or gain, heart problems, and circulatory disorders.

- **Thyroid problems:** The thyroid gland releases a special hormone called thyroxin that helps your metabolism to function properly. Sometimes a person's thyroid gland becomes overactive (hyperthyroidism), causing weight loss and rapid heartbeat, or underactive (hypothyroidism), causing weight gain, slower heart rate, and other bodily processes.

- **Metabolic syndrome:** This condition is diagnosed by the occurrence of three out of five of the following conditions: central trunk obesity, elevated blood pressure, elevated fasting glucose, high serum triglycerides, and low high-density cholesterol (also called high-density lipoprotein [HDL]) levels. Metabolic syndrome increases the risk of heart disease and diabetes. Some studies have estimated 34 percent of adults in the U.S. to have this syndrome. Most patients are older, obese, sedentary, and have some degree of insulin resistance. Stress can also be a contributing factor. The most important factors are genetics, diet (particularly sugar-sweetened beverage consumption), sedentary behavior, disrupted sleep, use of mood disorder medication, and excessive alcohol use.

Also, feminine health issues can wreak havoc with your metabolism:

- **Polycystic ovary syndrome (PCOS):** This is a condition characterized by excessive testosterone levels and lowered progesterone levels in women, leading to hairiness, irregular menstrual periods, problems with fertility, and weight gain due to insulin resistance. **TIP:** We have had great success with our clients who have PCOS when we put them on a dairy-free diet and add inositol, a powdered B vitamin that is also a sweetener and stool softener, to their smoothies. This is what inositol does for someone with PCOS:
  - increases progesterone
  - increases sex hormone binding globulin (SHBG), which deals with any free testosterone in the bloodstream
  - lowers testosterone levels
  - improves insulin sensitivity
  - decreases luteinizing hormone
  - induces weight loss
  - manages hirsutism
  - helps ovulation

- **Estrogen or testosterone dominance:** This hormonal problem can cause you to carry more weight for the same reasons as someone with PCOS. With extra testosterone or estrogen, you will retain more fluid and be more insulin resistant. If a doctor gives you a medication to fix one problem, it creates a domino effect with other problems, so this is a hard problem to correct. People with estrogen or testosterone dominance tend to carry a little extra weight and never reach their goal weight, no matter how hard they try.

Metabolic Tests

Do you feel that your metabolism is sluggish, but yet your thyroid tests always come back normal? Or perhaps you are on a synthetic hormone replacement, but you are still overweight and feel your metabolism is off?

At the Before and After Weight Loss Clinics, home of the Belly Buster Diet, we use a number of tests, written and otherwise, to determine how well your metabolism is working. Two of my favorites are the temperature test and this metabolic questionnaire. If your temperature is subnormal and your written score is high, call us and we can advise you about what your results mean. In some cases, we may suggest supplements that you can take to improve your metabolism. Our toll-free number is 1-888-657-5042.

1) Temperature Test

For ten days, take your temperature under your tongue, *before* you get out of bed. Record your temperature. Low basal temperature is one sign of poor thyroid function. If you have an average of less than 97.6 degrees over the ten days, are frequently fatigued, have a relative who has had a thyroid problem, and score high on the following test, chances are your body is making antibodies against your thyroid—even if your blood tests come back normal. If so, you could possibly benefit from a therapeutic dose of thyroid medication. **TIP:** Read *Thyroid Power: 10 Steps to Total Health* by Richard Shames and Karilee H. Shames and *Hypothyroidism, Health and Happiness* by Steven Hotze, MD. Both of these books are of enormous help in understanding how your thyroid works, and Hotze's book explains why lab tests may lie.

2) Written Metabolic Test

(Copy this to take the test or print it out if you are reading this online. You may want to take it to your doctor or reference it when calling us!)

Directions: Score each statement as follows:
10: This is a significant problem.
5: This is a problem but not a major issue.
2: This happens every now and then, but not often.
0: This seldom or never happens.

_____ 1) Do you have cold hands or feet?

_____ 2) Do you have swelling in the neck area?

_____ 3) Are you overweight? (Score 10 if 20 pounds overweight, 5 for 10 to 19 pounds, and 2 for 5 to 9 pounds.)

_____ 4) Can you eat very little and still not lose weight, or do you gain weight too easily?

_____ 5) Are you often tired?

_____ 6) Do you wake up with a heavy head or a headache that wears off as the day progresses?

_____ 7) Do you require a lot of sleep and still don't feel well rested?

_____ 8) Do you get tired during the day or feel an energy drop when you stop moving?

_____ 9) Does your energy drop significantly in the afternoon?

_____ 10) Do you rely on caffeine, nicotine, or some other stimulant to keep your energy going?

_____ 11) Women—Are your moods noticeably worse during your cycle?
Men—Do you lack a morning erection?

_____ 12) Do you have a short fuse (too easily irritable)?

_____ 13) Are you depressed, prone to depression, and/or do you feel less communicative or withdrawn?

_____ 14) Are you prone to depression in the fall or spring?

_____ 15) Is your memory noticeably declining?

_____ 16) Is the outside portion of your eyebrows thinning or gone?

_____ 17) Do you have dry skin or hair?

_____ 18) Do you have rough patches of skin on your elbows?

_____ 19) Is your body hair falling out, or do you have less body hair in general than you used to have?

_____ 20) Are you prone to constipation?

_____ 21) Do you have carpal tunnel syndrome or numbness in your extremities?

_____ 22) Are you prone to facial fluid retention, especially around the eyes?

_____ 23) Is your voice coarse or hoarse?

_____ 24) Do you have general muscle weakness or frequent muscle cramping?

_____ 25) Do you have high cholesterol, or low good cholesterol?

Total your answers. If your score is over 100, take this test to your doctor. You may have a hidden metabolic problem.

If your score is 50 to 100, your thyroid is struggling to function, and steps can be taken to significantly improve your health. Call Before and After Weight Loss Clinic at 1-888-657-5042 for a free metabolic assessment and see what we would recommend.

If your score is in the 20 to 49 range, you just need to take preventative steps to keep your health on track and cut down on the wear and tear.

If your score is under 20, your metabolism is in good condition.

TIP: We teach our clients not to eat foods that interfere with thyroxin output from the thyroid while they are losing weight. One of those foods is cabbage, which is ironic since everyone has heard of an unofficial plan, the cabbage soup diet. We replace cabbage with broccoli slaw. (It is right next to the bagged shredded cabbage in most grocery stores.) You can make coleslaw with it or stir-fries, but my favorite is this Chicken "Noodle" Soup. The strands of slaw become translucent like noodles.

Broccoli Slaw Chicken "Noodle" Soup
1 bag of broccoli slaw
1 cup of diced cooked chicken
1 carton of low sodium chicken broth
1 teaspoon Mrs. Dash

Mix all ingredients together in a saucepan and simmer until the strands are translucent. You may add other veggies, like string beans, broccoli florets, zucchini, or squash. Makes 4 servings.

TIP: Soy milk is preferable because it will not raise your blood sugar like dairy or almond. Contrary to myth, it will not affect your thyroid if you consume it in small amounts, but you should not take it within the time frame during which eating calcium is contraindicated with your thyroid medication. (You should stay away from processed soy, like bars and miso, but not soy milk.)

My Metabolic Score:_____

_____
_____
_____

24

3 WHAT SPEEDS UP YOUR METABOLISM?

What are you to do when your skinny best friend can inhale Dunkin' Donuts every morning and pizza every night and never gain an ounce, but you cannot look at 12 carbs without gaining 12 pounds? You can't change your age or your genetics; however, you can improve a few things, or at least do them differently. Sadly, they don't involve still eating donuts and pizza, but you will be happy that your metabolism improves. Here are eight things you can do to help immediately.

1) Breathe! Oxygen is the key to metabolism. You have to have oxygen to burn fat. The better you can oxygenate your body, the more efficiently you can speed up your metabolism and burn fat to lose weight. (On the other hand, try not breathing and see what happens!)

Try this right now: Put one hand on your chest and one on your stomach. What's happening? Not much! If there is hardly any movement, you're barely breathing—you're almost dead! Physiologists tell us that we use only about 20 percent of our lung capacity. They say that the majority of us are too tense to properly breathe and are barely breathing a large percentage of the time.

So you have two choices: You can work your butt off with aerobic exercise to aerate your body, or you can do simple breathing techniques fifteen minutes a day to aerate your body. If you picked aerobic exercise, find yourself a trainer and have fun doing it; all the busy people like me who hate to sweat, keep reading. These exercises cost you absolutely nothing, but are worth, oh, so much!

You can do this at specific times of the day when you are not doing anything else. For me, it is when I am riding the elevator, at stoplights on my way to and from work, or while watching television. Hold down one nostril and breathe in through the other as deeply as you can, filling your lungs so that your diaphragm rises as much as possible; hold it and count to ten. Then, let the air out slowly through your mouth. Repeat five times. Then repeat, holding down the other nostril. You may feel light-headed or slightly euphoric the first few times you do these breathing exercises. I have a friend who is an opera singer who lost 34 pounds when she learned these breathing techniques—without changing her eating habits!

2) Get seven to eight hours of sleep per night. Your body produces hormones while you sleep that help regulate your appetite and cravings. If you deprive your body of even a small portion of the sleep it needs, the important weight loss regulating hormones, such as insulin, leptin, and ghrelin, are thrown off and your chances of being heavier are greater. Sleeping seven to eight hours each night has been scientifically proven to increase your metabolism significantly.

3) Drink six to eight glasses of ice-cold water per day. German researchers have found that drinking lots of ice-cold water helps you have a higher metabolic rate. If you need to lose weight, the rule of thumb is eight 8-ounce glasses for the first 200 pounds and 8 ounces more for every 25 more pounds. So throw an ice cube in your pure water and enjoy an extra metabolic boost! In addition to its effect on your metabolic rate, sipping cold water throughout the day may cause you to eat less because your body usually doesn't distinguish hunger from thirst. Rather than reaching for a snack, you may feel satisfied with the water. **TIP:** When you think you are hungry, drink a glass of water first and wait awhile to see if it was really thirst.

4) Drink green tea. Green tea is naturally caffeinated and can stimulate your metabolism by up to 16 percent. It contains epigallocatechin gallate (EGCG), a chemical that stimulates the nervous system, increasing your heart and breathing rates. As a result, it revs up your metabolism and helps you burn calories faster. Green tea has flavonoids with fat-burning properties that also help with weight loss as well as many other health benefits.

TIP: If you don't like the taste, brew your own and mix it with Lipton black tea or other teas, like oolong tea, yerba mate, white tea, or matcha tea (a green tea that you don't have to brew that is excellent for weight loss). You can also use yacon syrup to sweeten it. A tablespoon of yacon syrup per day is good for weight loss also, but it is expensive. The syrup tastes like molasses and is a high-fiber sweetener with inulin that puts good bacteria in the gut and helps keep you regular.

5) Eat three meals per day, especially breakfast. When you skip a meal, your body goes into starvation mode and starts storing fat. If you are not feeding your body, it will conserve energy by slowing everything down so that your organs and your brain can keep functioning. To keep your metabolism high, you need to eat every four to five hours; and if you are hungry, you should have a protein snack in between.

Think of your food as fuel for your body much like wood burning in a campfire. The more logs you add to the campfire, the more that fire roars; but when you quit adding logs to the fire, what happens? The fire burns down to embers. If you don't consistently add logs, it can be hard to get the fire restarted. It is a lot easier to burn logs when that fire is stoked. Your body's metabolism is the same way; you have to feed it often so that your metabolic fire does not slow down.

6) Move! (OK, so maybe you should do a little more than just breathe!) If you like to exercise, good for you! If you don't, find something that you are willing to do. Some people join a gym, but it may not be for you. If you like to dance, take a course or perhaps do a video with exercise and dancing to music. If you like to walk, then either walk outdoors or on a treadmill indoors—put it in front of the TV if that is what it takes! During commercials, I put my laptop on the coffee table and go to the virtual gym on our clinic's website, http://bestdietsource.gostorego.com/gym.html, where we have partnered with FitStudio by Sears. FitStudio features Steve and Bonnie Pfiester, the national spokespersons for FitStudio by Sears and fitness professionals/owners of Max Fitness in Vero Beach, Florida, doing short video segments of different exercises. While you are watching the videos, you can work out with them!

You can also select exercise programs on the site to do on a more consistent basis. Check it out! FitStudio will even *pay* you each time you complete a workout with points you can turn into cash at Sears or Kmart! Isn't that a great incentive? Go to http://bestdietsource.gostorego.com/gym.html and check it out.

Walk, bike, swim, but find something that you are willing to do at least three times a week for at least twenty minutes to start and work up from there. Make a list *right now* of three things you are willing to do and start *this week*! Bottom line, you must move your body with some form of exercise to stimulate your metabolism and maximize the efforts of your diet plan.

7) Take probiotics and eat yogurt to help cleanse your gut. Researchers at Shanghai Jiao Tong University have reached an interesting conclusion that I have been hypothesizing for years: Obesity is due not only to overeating and a sedentary lifestyle, but also to the presence of a certain fat-boosting bacteria in the digestive tract. The researchers also found that diets that alter the mix of microorganisms in the gut can actually help you shed weight. According to the researchers, mice bred to be slim no matter what they ate became overweight when injected with a human bacteria called enterobacter and fed a rich diet. Enterobacter is found in high quantities in the guts of morbidly obese humans but not thin people, according to the *International Society for Microbial Ecology (ISME) Journal.*

When you eat a high-carbohydrate, high-fat diet (the opposite of the Before and After Belly Buster Diet) these bacteria leave the colon through the bloodstream and deposit in the fat cells in the abdomen. They cause a constant state of inflammation in the abdomen. It leads to glucose metabolism disorders like insulin resistance and metabolic syndrome, both of which are associated with obesity.

These findings are the latest evidence that microscopic gut bacteria play a role in human health and that adding yogurt and other probiotic foods to your diet can alter bacterial cultures in the human digestive tract and reduce the risks of obesity, diabetes, and other health problems. The human digestive tract is home to billions of bacteria, some of which are helpful and some of which are harmful to our health. Probiotics are normal bacteria that exist in your colon to aid digestion and regulation of your immune system—and now it's clear they help you lose weight. If you like yogurt, then incorporate it into your diet at least three to four times per week for breakfast or as a snack, and take probiotics as a supplement for a few weeks every few months (we carry them on our website, http://www.bestdietsource.com/. If you don't like yogurt or you are lactose intolerant, bitter melon can also kill off the bad bacteria and preserve the good bacteria. Bitter melon is an ingredient found in our appetite suppressants. Drinking green tea and white tea is also helpful. The herb curcumin (curry powder) and quercetin (a flavonoid found in berries and many other foods) also protect the good bacteria and don't kill the bad.

Eating yogurt would be a way to enjoy a calcium-rich food while using a probiotic. Here is a recipe with yogurt that can be used for breakfast or for a snack:

Yogurt Parfait
1 6-ounce Dannon Light & Fit Carb & Sugar Control Yogurt
¼ cup Mona's Granola (original)
¼ cup blueberries (or any fruit)
1 tablespoon Cool Whip (optional)

Greek yogurt with fruit tastes so decadent; however, if you read the label, most brands contain 22 or more grams of carbohydrates. That is not so good for your diet, despite the fact that Greek yogurt contains more protein. So what's a dieting gal to do when she really loves the taste of a good, pudding-y (I made up that word) Greek yogurt? Try plain Chobani Greek yogurt. It has only 7 grams of carbohydrates and 18 grams of protein. You can add fruit to plain Chobani and make up your own recipes, but I will share a few of mine here. The best thing to do when dieting is use the Dannon Light & Fit Carb & Sugar Control Yogurt which has 3 grams of carbohydrates and 60 calories, or the 80-calorie Dannon Light & Fit. Try mixing in a tablespoon of plain Chobani and freeze it for ten minutes. The whole thing tastes amazingly like Greek yogurt when you put just a little in, and it saves some calories, carbs, and money!

Here are ten of my favorite yogurt ideas:
1) Make a parfait: Mix 2 tablespoons each of half Greek yogurt and half Dannon Light & Fit Carb & Sugar Control Yogurt and put it over ¼ cup of Mona's Granola. Top with ½ cup of any kind of berries (I love the mixed berries from Sam's

Club) and 1 tablespoon of whipped cream.

2) Make pumpkin pudding by mixing 2 tablespoons of canned pumpkin with 3 tablespoons of plain yogurt and sweeten to taste with Wisdom Natural Brands SweetLeaf Sweet Drops in English Toffee flavor.

3) Make frozen yogurt by adding egg whites and sweetener to plain yogurt. Put it in the freezer and stir every thirty minutes until frozen. My favorite is made with pureed peaches. I use one container (6 ounces) of Chobani, ¼ cup egg whites, and 1/3 cup peaches.

4) Make a gelatin mousse by dividing a batch of sugar-free gelatin in half; add plain yogurt to half and pour it into a glass dish. Pour the rest of the plain gelatin on top and refrigerate. It's good two-toned or scrambled together. You can do colors for teams or holidays.

5) Use plain yogurt to make tartar sauce by adding pickles and dill weed.

6) Make a great tzatziki sauce for turkey burgers by adding shredded cucumbers and garlic to yogurt.

7) Use yogurt to coat chicken before cooking in the skillet or slow cooker. I especially like it before breading it with panko and Tajin or making a tandoori dish. It is also good with lemon pepper seasoning.

8) Yogurt smoothies are thick and yummy with this rich pudding. Try mixing 3 ounces of yogurt, 4 ounces of soy milk, and 4 ounces of water with a teaspoon of sugar-free gelatin (or a packet of gelatin protein powder) and a handful of frozen fruit in a blender.

9) Make a soup with 3 ounces of yogurt, 4 ounces of creamed broccoli or creamed cauliflower, and 8 ounces of low-sodium chicken broth. Top with grated cheese and a little grated carrot.

10) Use Chobani yogurt to make ranch dressing. I really missed my ranch dressing on low-carb diets because I could not find one I liked.

Ranch Dressing
2 containers (12 ounces) Chobani plain yogurt
1 envelope Hidden Valley Ranch mix

½ cup skim milk or soy milk (I like mine thick so I use a little less milk)

Mix all ingredients in a mason jar and refrigerate.
Serving size: 2 tablespoons (16 servings)
Protein: 2.5 grams
Carbs: 1.3 grams
Fat: .1 grams

8) Remember milky, spicy, fishy, and nutty. These foods have been shown to increase metabolism:

- calcium-rich foods
- spicy foods
- foods high in omega-3 fatty acids
- foods with arginine

Let's look at each one to see how you could incorporate them into your diet.

Calcium-Rich Foods
Research has shown that calcium intake can speed up weight loss by as much as 67 percent while eating a low-fat diet. Adding a calcium supplement *and* eating calcium-rich foods would ensure that you are getting an abundance of calcium to do the job. If you don't like milk, other calcium-rich foods are available.

Look for fat-free or low-fat milk products. (Lactose-reduced milk products are also good sources of calcium. If you are lactose intolerant, take Lactaid or Dairy Aid—this is too important to miss out on!) Here are some options:

- fat-free or low-fat yogurt
- fat-free or low-fat (1 percent) milk
- soy milk or almond milk fortified with calcium (not flavored)
- low-fat cheese (3 grams of fat or less per serving)
- fat-free or low-fat cottage cheese

These green vegetables are also a great way to get calcium:

- turnip greens
- kale

- broccoli
- collard greens

Fresh is preferable, but if you do buy canned vegetables, look for the ones labeled "low sodium" or "no salt added". If you buy frozen foods, choose ones without sauces.

Smoothies make great, calcium-filled, mid-morning or mid-afternoon snacks. They are quick to make with a Magic Bullet or a counter-top blender—you can't beat an Osterizer for making smoothies. (There are many smoothie recipes are listed on our blog, www.bellybusterbabe.blogspot.com.) Smoothies can be made with protein powders, fruit, gelatin, low-fat puddings, yogurt, chocolate, and even vegetables. You can mix in eggs or Egg Beaters, flavorings, and extracts. Add ground flaxseed meal or ground walnuts for a nutty flavor. Frozen fruits like strawberries, blueberries, raspberries, pineapple, and peaches make a thicker smoothie. For most smoothies, I use about one cup of liquid (½ water and ½ soy milk) and a cup of ice. You can add gelatin or a protein supplement or powdered peanut butter to thicken it. If you are in the maintenance phase of your diet, you can use 1 to 2 tablespoons of frozen dairy-free desserts to your protein shakes to thicken them after adding fruit. Choose from products like So Delicious Dairy Free coconut milk or soy milk frozen desserts, Almond Dream frozen dessert, or Arctic Zero. Walden Farms sugar-free, fat-free chocolate syrup and caramel dip, and PB2, a low-fat powdered peanut butter with 85 percent less fat, are also great to have on hand and can be ordered on our website, www.bestdietsource.com.

Spice it Up! Hot! Hot! Hot!
Would you like a great way to increase your metabolism by 25 percent for the next couple of hours? You can do it daily if you wish! Yes, it really is possible—just eat something spicy!

Hot peppers in spicy foods will increase your heart rate and raise your body temperature. Capsaicin, the substance that gives peppers their hotness, can speed up metabolism by up to 25 percent for three hours or so and can help you burn more than 300 extra calories per day without any extra effort. According to the *New York Times*, research has also shown that people who use hot pepper sauce consume an average of 200 fewer calories throughout the day.

If you don't care for spicy foods, I know how you feel—I didn't either, until I realized I could use them to my advantage. My suggestion would be to start out with small amounts and build up to bolder amounts. I now make my own turkey sausage and put pepper flakes in the patties—a lot more than before! And I use Spice Hunter Thai seasoning. It is delicious in stir-fries. I started with a pinch, and now I use a whole teaspoonful. One of our Spanish clients introduced me to Tajin seasoning, which is a mild chili with lime crystals. Tajin is divine on fish, chicken, and even melons or potatoes. She also told me about Valentina picante sauce and ketchup. It is a little hot for me now, so I mix it with my Walden Farms Ketchup. But I am working up to having it straight from the bottle!

Hot wings was one of the things I missed most on low-fat diets. During the Super Bowl, I didn't want to be left out and discovered a wonderful recipe that you can make as hot as you want. It really tastes like chicken wings! You can find it on our clinics' blog with a lot other low-fat, low-carb recipes at www.bellybusterbabe.blogspot.com, and you can find the products to make it on our website, www.bestdietsource.com.

Buffalo Chicken Dip
1 large can of white chunk chicken
1 jar of Walden Farms fat-free ranch or bleu cheese dip
1 cup of Walden Farms fat-free, calorie-free
   original barbeque sauce
8 ounces fat-free cream cheese
1 cup grated sharp cheddar cheese
1/4 cup chopped spring onions
Add celery sticks for dipping
   (and tortilla chips for those not dieting)

Mix the dip and sauce with the softened cream cheese in a 9x13 glass dish. Stir in the chicken chunks. Top with grated cheese and bake at 350° for 20 minutes. Top with onions, if desired. Serve with celery sticks for dieters and Tostidos or tortilla chips for non-dieters. Add a dash of Tabasco sauce or wing sauce if you want it hotter.

Before you decide you just can't stomach spicy foods, read on: Contrary to the popular belief that ulcer sufferers should avoid spicy foods, a report published in *Digestive Diseases and Sciences* concluded that capsaicin increased blood flow in the stomach's mucous lining, which may help in healing of the stomach tissue. Capsaicin also protects against the side effects of aspirin, and chili pepper eaters develop fewer peptic ulcers than those who eat plain foods. The rates of stomach cancer are unusually low in countries where chili peppers are a regular part of the diet, as capsaicin appears to neutralize some carcinogens.

Perhaps the best arguments for adding hot peppers as a spice to your diet are these two points: 1) Chili peppers are an incredible replacement for the fat and salt in your diet, as the flavors of the foods are enhanced enough that you won't miss the fat and salt; and 2) medical studies have shown that capsaicin significantly lowers cholesterol and can help ward off strokes and heart attacks.

Pass the Prilosec; I am eating more chili!

TIP: Speaking of chili, most chili recipes call for beans, all of which have a lot of carbs. To cut the overall carb count in your chili but still get the metabolic boost from the chili peppers, add some quartered button mushrooms. The seasonings will flavor them, and you won't be able to tell the difference in the texture or the taste.

Lee's Low-Carb Beanless Chili
½ pound lean ground beef, turkey, or chicken
1 jar of Classico Spicy Red Pepper pasta sauce
  (or make your own)
1 large ripe tomato, diced (*not* canned)
1 pint button mushrooms, quartered
1 teaspoon chili powder
¼ teaspoon Tabasco sauce
1/2 cup grated sharp cheddar cheese
1/4 cup chopped spring onions

Brown the meat in a skillet and add the chili powder. Place the tomato sauce in a saucepan and add the diced tomato, then add the browned meat and quartered mushrooms. Simmer for about 30 minutes until mushrooms have cooked well. Add Tabasco sauce to taste. Serve with cheese and onions on top. You may serve over a salad for a taco salad, or if you are maintaining your weight, serve with a small amount of Fritos corn chips.

TIP: Add a packet of protein soup to a cup of chili or any kind of meat sauce and you will eat much less.

Another spicy food known for being a metabolism booster is ginger; it's also known for having a soothing affect on the bowels. Eating a dish with ground or sliced ginger can speed up the metabolic rate as much as 20 percent. Fresh ginger is great with seafood and stir-fries as well as dissolved in teas. Wasabi and ginger on sushi are both doing more than pleasing and tingling your palate!

Fish and other Sources of Omega-3

The American Heart Association has recommended eating fish high in omega-3 fatty acids one to two times a week to prevent heart attacks. Did you know that they also help improve your metabolism? Researchers from the University of Western Ontario report that docosahexaenoic acid (DHA) and eicosapentaenoic acid (EPA), the omega-3 fatty acids found only in fish oil, can dramatically boost your metabolism by about 400 calories per day. Fish oil increases levels of fat-burning enzymes and decreases levels of fat-storage enzymes in your body. The fishes highest in omega-3 are salmon, tuna, trout, and halibut. (Anchovies and sardines are high in omega-3, but those are not right for dieting.) For the best metabolism-boosting benefit, you may also choose capsules containing at least 300 total milligrams of EPA and DHA. We sell them online as EFA, or Essential Fatty Acids; 1000 milligrams contains EPA, DHA, and conjugated linoleic acid (CLA) from a fish source to increase fat-burning and protect your heart.

Here is my favorite fish recipe. Fish like mahi-mahi, tilapia, snapper, or any kind of whitefish works well in this dish. It incorporates orange juice, which is high in calcium and omega-3, and nuts and fish, both of which have omega-3 oils.

Favorite Floridian Fish Recipe

4 fish fillets
1 cup orange juice
1 egg or ¼ cup Egg Beaters

½ cup unsalted shelled pistachios, crushed
1 teaspoon salt-free Mrs. Dash

Soak the fillets overnight in orange juice. Roll the fillets in egg, then season with Mrs. Dash. Then roll in nuts and bake on a tin-foil lined baking sheet at 350° for 10 minutes. Note: If you don't have enough nuts to coat all the filets, coat in crushed Melba toast or panko crumbs first and then put the nuts on top.

TIP: Eat seafood and fish when you eat out if you don't enjoy cooking it. Just make sure it isn't fried or loaded with butter so that you can keep your promise to yourself and meet your goal!

Since nuts are a great source of omega-3 fatty acids, incorporate them into foods in creative ways (on some diet plans, you may have to wait until a certain phase).

- stir-fries with cashews or almonds
- salads topped with walnuts
- pesto sauce made with ground walnuts
- baked chicken or trout with toasted almonds
- baked okra with pumpkin seeds (very low-carb!)

Besides the fish and nuts mentioned, these foods are also very high in omega-3 fatty acids:

- soy milk
- edamame
- eggs
- flaxseed
- spinach
- walnuts
- canola oil
- margarine made from soybeans
- protein supplements for weight loss

TIP: For an extra fat-burning boost, put a half to 2 teaspoons of ground flaxseed meal in your smoothies. The meal gives it a wonderful nutty taste, and it helps keep you regular! You can also add a half teaspoon of powdered inositol. It is a natural sweetener and will also soften your stool. Use more inositol if you have PCOS (see http://www.pcosdietsupport.com) or need to increase your progesterone (menopause) or have an excess of testosterone.

Sources of the Amino Acid Arginine

Flaxseed, nuts, and fish are also rich in arginine. According to a study in the *Journal of Nutrition*, the addition of arginine to the diet promotes the oxidation of fat and glucose and increases lean muscle. Researchers added arginine to the diets of obese mice in the study over a three-month period, and their body fat substantially decreased. This amino acid is particularly high in watermelon, but it is found in higher quantities in seafood, nuts, and seeds. Although watermelon has a high glycemic value, we have included it on the Belly Buster Diet for occasional consumption because of its high arginine content. (If you have IBS, be aware that watermelon could cause cramping and may not be a fruit you should choose; see chapter eight "Food Allergies, Irritable Bowel Syndrome, and Gluten Sensitivity".) Powdered peanut butter, PB2, is also great source of arginine and may be incorporated in your smoothies and used for snacks.

What is the most important thing that you will change to help your metabolism and your current weight issues?

_____

_____

_____

_____

_____

_____

_____

_____

_____

_____

NOTES:_____

_____

_____

_____

_____

_____

_____

_____

_____

_____

_____

_____

_____

_____

_____

_____

_____

_____

_____

_____

_____

_____

_____

_____

4 WHAT SLOWS DOWN YOUR METABOLISM?

We all know that inactivity and hypothyroidism slows your metabolism down, but what about alcohol, stress, and preservatives in foods? How badly does each of those actually affect us? Also, what about inflammation in the body? Inflammation can also be caused from infection, illness, and compromised body function, even obesity, and you may not even know you have it. For instance, a medical situation like a heart attack or a severe infection of an organ may be looming and your body uses its energy and secretes special chemicals to fight it, unbeknownst to you, slowing down your metabolism. Certain foods you eat can cause inflammation also.

Alcohol
Why is it more difficult to lose weight while drinking alcohol? Alcohol, even hard liquor, contains calories and has other effects on your appetite that may interfere with your weight loss efforts. First of all, an ounce of hard liquor (gin, vodka, rum, whiskey, or scotch) contains 64 calories for 80 proof varieties and 80 calories for those that are 100 proof. (The proof refers to the percentage of alcohol in the liquor: 80 proof is 40 percent alcohol; 100 proof is 50 percent alcohol.) If you drink three to four drinks, they could be

contributing anywhere from 192 to 320 calories—and that's if you're using only one ounce per drink. Many drinks at bars or made at home are made with more than an ounce. If you're also adding a mixer, the calories may soar! Consider that, per 8-ounce cup, orange juice contains 111 calories, regular cola, or lemon-lime soda pop has about 100 calories, and regular ginger ale or tonic water has around 80 calories. If you drink mixed drinks, you can easily take in over 500 calories per day from your libations. For an average-sized, moderately active woman, that's about a third of her minimum total daily intake of 1,600 to 2,400 calories.

In addition to the calories, when a person drinks, alcohol takes preference. The liver breaks down alcohol for energy first, causing a buildup of fatty acids. What this means is that when you drink alcohol, the body uses the calories supplied from alcohol before it is able to expend the calories from fat. This characteristic is referred to as "fat sparing," meaning that alcohol's presence spares the fat from being utilized for energy. Alcohol also stimulates appetite in many people. It also lowers your inhibitions to the point you may not care that you have a goal that was so important to you before you imbibed. This may thwart your weight loss efforts even more.

Alcohol can add empty calories to your daily nutrition and it can jeopardize your health. Alcohol influences your nutritional status, affecting the hormones responsible for fluid balance. When drinking alcohol, people tend to urinate more frequently, losing body fluids, and they can become dehydrated and thirsty. It becomes a vicious cycle because the only way to break the cycle is to have water or another non-alcoholic beverage. Along with the fluids drinkers lose, they excrete important nutrients as well: calcium, magnesium, potassium, and zinc. Alcohol also interferes with the absorption of vitamins B1 (thiamin), B6, B12, and folic acid. It causes problems in processing vitamins A and D, too. As a result, people who drink in excess often have nutritional deficiencies.

The following chart gives you an idea of the calories present in alcoholic beverages:

BEVERAGE	SERVING (ounces)	PROOF (percent alcohol)	CALORIES
Beer, regular	12	10 to 12 proof (5 to 6 percent)	150
Beer, light	12	8 to 10 proof (4 to 5 percent)	105
Wine	4	24 proof (12 percent)	77
Wine cooler	10	10 to 13 proof (5 to 6.5 percent)	125
Vodka, gin, rum, whiskey, or scotch	1	80 proof (40 percent) 100 proof (50 percent)	64 (80 proof) 80 (100 proof)
Cordials, liqueurs	1	32 to 52 proof (16 to 26 percent)	103 to 123

Recent research has shown that alcohol may increase HDL, the "good" cholesterol that gives protective benefits from heart disease. On the other hand, a 2002 report published by the *British Medical Journal* found that the benefits and risks of drinking alcohol vary by age and sex. It's also worth remembering that the risk of death from diseases, including many types of cancer (colon, breast, liver, and oral), hypertension, liver disease, and heart disease is also linked with alcohol consumption. The greater the amount of alcohol a woman drinks, particularly at a younger age, the greater the likelihood of death from one of the above-mentioned diseases.

This latest study also shows that the risks of these conditions are lowest for nondrinkers under the age of 35, for both men and women. For 16- to 24-year-olds, risks increase when women drink more than eight drinks per week and when men drink more than five drinks per week. Risks also increase with age when women have eight to twenty drinks a week, and when men have five to thirty-four drinks a week. In most cases, the negatives greatly outweigh the positives, particularly if you are attempting to lose weight.

If you would like to cut back on your alcohol consumption to make losing weight easier, first examine your own drinking patterns. Ask yourself questions like:

- What does drinking three to four drinks of hard liquor or wine every day offer me?
- What might happen if I cut down to one drink a day, or gradually limit myself to three to four throughout the week or just on special occasions?
- What is encouraging me to lose weight?
- Might a desire to be healthier motivate me to modulate my drinking?
- Is drinking necessary at all?

TIP: I switched to spritzers at first and then gradually quit drinking while dieting. I learned to make delicious virgin smoothies that I enjoy just as much, if not more, without the alcohol. The calories and the struggle for my liver to burn fat are just not worth it to me.

Virgin Piña Colada Shake
2/3 cup water
1 packet Before and After vanilla crème pudding or banana pudding
or 1 scoop of vanilla protein
½ cup naturally sweetened crushed pineapple, drained
½ teaspoon coconut flavoring (I like the Watkins brand)
½ teaspoon banana flavoring
½ teaspoon rum flavoring (optional)
1 cup ice

Put all ingredients, except ice, in blender and blend. Then crush ice into the mixture.

Virgin White Russian

You can make this several ways: cold or hot; with soy or almond milk; with coffee and a diet cappuccino mix; or with pudding and a cappuccino mix.

1 packet Before and After vanilla crème pudding mix, or 1
  scoop of vanilla protein
1 packet Before and After cappuccino mix
  or 1 scoop of mocha or cappuccino protein mix
1 cup of ice
1 cup of water
2 ounces coffee (optional)

Blend in a blender that has an ice crusher setting.

This is my favorite, and I could swear it has vodka in it! It tastes like a mudslide when you add a tablespoon of Walden Farms chocolate sauce. You can add half the water and add ½ cup soy or almond milk instead. On maintenance phases, you can add 2 tablespoons of a frozen nondairy dessert to make it thicker and creamier for a fantastic frappuccino .

Stress

Do you do pretty well on your diet until the first emotional crisis, and then the stress drives you straight to the desserts? Stress seems to permeate every facet of our lives these days. Unfortunately, the overproduction of the stress hormone, cortisol, can wreak havoc in your body. Cortisol is a hormone that has several uses that are crucial to proper functioning of your body. Released by the adrenal glands (located just above your kidneys) during times of stress, cortisol has several functions in the body, including blood pressure regulation, glucose mobilization, and the reduction of inflammation. It gives you a quick burst of adrenaline if you need a to respond to a stressful situation. It also decreases your pain, heightens your memory, and helps maintain a healthy balance of other hormones in your body. Therefore, you have to have some cortisol present; however, chronically high levels of cortisol can impede overall health.

Excess cortisol levels can cause fatigue, fat accumulation in the tummy, and decreased immunity. Permanently high cortisol levels can cause adrenal fatigue. Raised cortisol levels eventually lead to sudden weight gain, muscle degeneration, blood sugar imbalances, a decrease in bone density, and an inability to concentrate. Eventually the body's relaxation response never kicks in due to repeated cortisol production.

Overproduction can lead to cortisol bottoming out and becoming low, leading to a dangerous situation. Low cortisol levels are the result of the body's production slowing down due to flooding and overuse. The body no longer has the proper "fight or flight" response, and reaction times to stressful situations are severely slowed. Both conditions affect your weight and fat accumulation.

The key to losing weight is to have all of your hormones working together toward that goal. If you have excess cortisol in your bloodstream, losing weight can be extremely difficult. Here are tips to get your cortisol under control:

- A healthy diet, regular exercise, and a regimented eight hours of sleep are three key secrets to balancing your cortisol levels.

- Oxygenate your body to help you relax and lower cortisol levels. At every stop light and during commercials (if you watch TV), hold one nostril closed and breathe in deeply through the other, feeling your diaphragm lift—take in as much air as your lungs will hold. Count to ten and release through your mouth. Do 5 times through each nostril.

- Avoid stress and do yoga, meditation, and/or affirmations. Affirm that you are calm, cool, and collected at all times, in every situation. My favorite mantra is, "Everything turns out exquisitely, better than I could have ever planned it." God has a plan for you, and it is a good plan. (See chapter eighteen "How to Do Affirmations.)

- Eat the foods that research shows can help lower cortisol levels in the body. Here are ten foods that help lower your cortisol levels and therefore help get rid of dreaded belly fat:

1) black tea
2) fish oil (omega-3 rich foods include halibut, and salmon) and canola oil
3) liver, grilled
4) citrus fruits (oranges, grapefruits, limes, lemons)
5) bell peppers (if you have IBS, do red only)

6) dark chocolate (40 grams per day; use unsweetened in smoothies while dieting)
7) nuts like walnuts
8) seeds like flaxseed and chia seed
9) yogurt and ricotta cheese
10) soybeans

Here is a menu for lowering cortisol after a day of unbearable stress:

<u>Breakfast:</u>
Mona's Granola topped with 2 ounces of walnuts
1 tub of light yogurt
hot tea

<u>Midmorning:</u>
1/2 grapefruit (try heating it in the microwave with a little brown sugar and honey) or orange or tangerine

<u>Lunch:</u>
iced tea
drizzle yogurt and lime juice over salad:
   dark green lettuces
   bell pepper
   tangerine slices
   2 ounces walnuts
      blueberries or strawberries
      salmon
   steamed broccoli

<u>Midafternoon:</u>
orange
2 squares of 70 percent dark chocolate bar

<u>Dinner:</u>
liver and onions
steamed cauliflower
bell pepper
tomato
toasted 40-calorie bread

After dinner:
decaf hot black tea

Stressed spelled backwards is *desserts!* Do you blow your diet on desserts a couple of times a week or do you have a plan in place to help you with those sweet cravings? Do you get in enough fruit that you feel like your need for sugar is satisfied? Do you reach for food when you are in a crisis? Let's come up with a plan.

The first plan of action for changing your diet is to banish the cookies, cake, and the high-carb junk food from your house. If you have others in your household who are not dieting and you cannot stay away from their junk food, consider getting a separate small refrigerator for them and a big plastic tub or sweater container for the closet or pantry. Out of sight will be out of mind for you. Replace those things with both fresh and frozen fruits. Make desserts from those.

From fourteen years of observing food journals in my clinics, I believe one reason most people eat too many sweets is that they don't consume enough fruit. Here are ten simple diet-friendly desserts, some with fruit and some without. Keep the list on the refrigerator so you will think before you grab! These desserts are all simple to make and you can use them on most any diet.

1) Sugar-free gelatin with a dollop of Cool Whip. **TIP:** Use real whipped cream or Reddi-wip if you prefer but only 1 to 2 tablespoons at a time; use regular Cool Whip, not light or fat-free—it is a marketing ploy and they have roughly the same fat grams with not near the taste, and they have hydrogenated oils that you may want to avoid. As far as sugar-free gelatin, it does not contain that much aspartame; but if you are allergic or want to avoid it all together, you can make your own gelatin like I do. You simply use one packet of Knox gelatin and 1 to 2 cups of sugar-free drink sweetened with Stevia or sucralose, like Kool-Aid. Make your own flavors and add fruit if you like.

2) Low-fat Light n' Lively cottage cheese with crushed pineapple and blueberries. Add nuts, like pecans or walnuts, if you are on a diet that allows them.

3) A frozen fruit smoothie with sugar-free gelatin and low-carb milk, soy milk, or almond milk. You can use frozen

peaches, berries, cherries, or pineapple.

4) Fruit trifle with blackberries, strawberries, peaches, and blueberries. (Cool Whip optional.)
5) Sugar-free popsicles.
6) Chocolate honey graham cracker, Melba toast, or celery with PB2 (powdered peanut butter has only 1.5 g fat versus 16 g fat in regular peanut butter). **TIP:** PB2 is sweeter if you mix it with a teaspoon of Walden Farms marshmallow dip.
7) Walden Farms fat-free sugar-free caramel dip with a half of an apple or Walden Farms chocolate dip with a cup of strawberries. (Walden Farms and PB2 products are available on our website at www.bestdietsource.com.)
8) Baked egg custard with eggs, milk, sweetener, and pudding mix (see our blog for complete recipe www.bellybusterbabe.blogspot.com)
9) Pumpkin pie with eggs, milk, and pumpkin (see our blog for complete recipe: www.bellybusterbabe.blogspot.com)
10) Cheesecake made of cottage cheese or no-fat cream cheese (see blog, http://www.bellybusterbabe.blogspot.com/). We have recipes for amaretto, mocha, triple chocolate, strawberry, lime, orange, pineapple upside-down, and cappuccino coffee cake. (There are more cheesecake recipes in chapter six, "Diet-Friendly Substitutions.")

For more menus, diet plans, and low-calorie dessert ideas for those stressed-out days, please call Before and After Weight Loss Clinics for an appointment at 1-888-657-5042 or go to www.beforeandafterdiet.net or http://www.bestdietsource.com and fill out your health profile for a free metabolic assessment. We have clients on the Belly Buster Diet all over the US and Canada!

Preservatives

Preservatives slow down your metabolism, so it is better to eat everything fresh and natural and nothing out of a box or a can when you are trying to lose weight. In this age of Hamburger Helper and frozen TV dinners, people think they are saving time and money using the prepackaged foods. Do you really think "healthy" frozen dinners will help you lose weight? Well, think again!

Many of my clients come in and say that they have been dieting, but when I ask them about what they've been eating, a mainstay of their diet seems to be the frozen dinners that you buy at the grocer. In case you haven't read the labels, I will post some of them here for you. If the fat or the carbohydrates don't get you, the sodium usually does. And on top of that, all of them have lots of preservatives! Preservatives are additives that extend a food's shelf life. They prevent the spoilage of food from bacteria, molds, and fungi by slowing down changes in color and texture that make the food inedible or unappetizing. They will also slow down your weight loss.

Almost all frozen dinners are high in fat, carbs, sodium, or all three. You can make you own frozen dinners, as I will show you; but first, let's see what else is in the more popular frozen dinners in addition to preservatives that can slow down your weight loss.

Healthy Choice Oven-Roasted Chicken
Fat: 5 grams
Carbs: 33 grams
Sodium: 530 grams
Calories: 240

Weight Watchers Chicken Parmesan
Fat: 7 grams
Carbs: 40 grams
Sodium: 680 grams
Calories: 320

Lean Cuisine Baked Chicken with Stuffing and Potatoes
Fat: 7 grams
Carbs: 30 grams
Sodium: 600 grams
Calories: 240
(Not bad, but high glycemic

All of these are too high in carbohydrates for a low-carb diet, and they're high in sodium. Beef dishes were actually slightly lower in fat and carbs, but no better with sodium. We also found you do not get a satisfying amount of beef in them.

You would think seafood frozen dinners would be healthy, but they are either breaded or have sauce with it—and up go the carbs.

Healthy Choice Lemon Pepper Fish
(comes with rice, broccoli, and apple dessert)
Fat: 4 grams
Carbs: 58 grams
Sodium: 480 grams
Calories: 330 grams
(The salt and fat levels are great, but the carbs are quadruple what you need.)

Lean Cuisine Shrimp and Angel Hair Pasta
Fat: 4 grams
Carbs: 34 grams
Sodium: 610 grams
Calories: 230

TIP: The reason so many people use frozen dinners is because it is a quick way to prepare dinner, but I promise: You will not lose weight using store-bought frozen dinners! Instead, take one afternoon a month to make your own. If you freeze your own dinners, they will have a lot less sodium, carbs, and calories and taste much fresher. We share many more casserole and quiche recipes with our clients, but we follow the same basic recipe that I am going to share with you here.

Take a Sunday afternoon (or any day where you have a couple of hours to prepare your freezer meals) to do this. Use freezer-to-oven/microwave containers to make your concoctions. I like to use 8x8 Pyrex containers. I bake several on the same day and freeze them. At any given time, I have a chicken and broccoli, shrimp creole, vegetable lasagna, and diet chicken potpie to choose from in my freezer. I score them before freezing so servings easily pop out of the frozen dish for microwaving.

This is the basic casserole recipe:
1) Spray an 8x8 dish with a cooking spray.
2) Crumble 4 pieces of toasted 40- or 45-calorie bread or 12 pieces of crushed Melba toast in the bottom of the dish. If you are on a gluten-free diet, use toasted Rudi's gluten-free bread.

3) Place 4 servings of shredded meat on top of the crushed toast. You can use beef, ground turkey, chicken, shrimp, or pork. I use 12 ounces, but if your menu calls for 4 ounces per dinner meal, you will quadruple that serving to equal 16 ounces. However, if you add 4 ounces of cheese on the top of the casserole, deduct 4 ounces of meat to allow for the extra protein.

4) You may use any vegetable of your choice on top of the meat, as long as it is on your diet plan. I use 12 ounces of vegetables.

5) Pour low-sodium cream soup over the mixture. I use 2 to 4 packets of our protein soup from our site.

6) Top with 4 ounces grated cheese (optional).

Creole Casserole
4 pieces of 40-calorie bread, toasted
1 small bag of frozen shrimp or 2 cups fresh shrimp
1½ diced tomatoes,
   or 1 jar Classico Spicy Red Pepper pasta sauce
½ red or green bell pepper
chopped onion (or scallions) to taste
chili powder to taste
2 to 4 packets of Before and After protein tomato
   soup mix (optional)
   (use only 2 if you use the Classico sauce)
4 ounces Swiss cheese, grated
Follow directions above for the basic casserole.

Preservatives are in more foods, of course, than just frozen dinners. With the exception of unprocessed, organic fresh produce, just about all food is treated with some kind of preservative. Drinks, baked goods, milk, meats, cereals, candy, fruit, vegetables, oils and margarines, and all packaged or canned goods are all likely to contain some form of preservative unless advertised as preservative-free. Look for the names of the most common food preservatives on product labels: sodium benzoate, BHA, BHT, EDTA, tocopherols (vitamin E), calcium propionate, sodium nitrite, calcium sorbate, or potassium sorbate. The fewer processed foods with preservatives you can do while dieting, the easier it will be. It will also be easier to maintain your weight when you stay away from those additives.

Inflammation and C-Reactive Protein

Scientists have learned that imbalances in your diet can lead to the creation of excessive amounts of inflammatory chemicals called prostaglandins, and that can lead to an increase in your body's inflammatory response. Conversely, the consumption of certain nutrients allows your body to produce more anti-inflammatory prostaglandins, which can reduce inflammation. This is important when you are losing weight because when your body is fighting inflammation, your metabolism is not functioning optimally. Your body is using some of its energy to fight the inflammation, rather than to lose the weight.

According to William Joel Meggs, who is part of the toxicology department at Brody School of Medicine at East Carolina University, uncontrolled inflammation is a component of heart disease, lupus, arthritis, atherosclerosis, asthma, Alzheimer's, and many other ailments, including obesity.

Inflammation is not always as obvious as the above examples. It can silently involve every cell in your body and, over time, negatively affect your health and abilities. For example, allergies, joint pain, and premature aging are just a few of the common ailments linked to systemic inflammation.

But if you can't see inflammation, how do you measure it? Just like prostaglandins, other chemicals increase with increased levels of inflammation and can be measured. One of these chemical markers is a protein called C-reactive protein (CRP). CRP is often measured in conjunction with other blood tests, and normal values are well established. From a clinical standpoint, a CRP level of less than 5 milligrams per liter of blood is considered normal. "Normal" may not be optimal, however, for losing weight. Many medical researchers believe that even the slightest elevations of CRP are tied to increased risk for heart attack, stroke, and even obesity. If you'd like to have your CRP measured, consult your physician, who can order a simple blood test.

A registered dietitian and a food chemist chose all anti-inflammatory foods for both our diet and our maintenance plan on the Belly Buster Diet. Some other places to find lists of anti-inflammatory foods are in William Meggs' book, *The Inflammation Cure*, and Monica Reinagel's *The Inflammation Free Diet Plan*.

Here is my top-ten list of anti-inflammatory foods:
1. **Salmon:** Cold-water fish contain omega-3 oils, and wild salmon has more than farmed-raised.
2. **Grass-fed beef:** This has omega-3s but not as much as fish, and grain-fed beef has virtually none.
3. **Cherries:** A study in the *Journal of Nutrition* showed that eating cherries significantly reduced inflammation. They are also packed with antioxidants and are relatively low in calories and low on the glycemic index.
4. **Blueberries:** Frozen blueberries are just as good as fresh and have all the natural compounds that will reduce inflammation.
5. **Ginger:** Brew your own ginger tea by peeling several thin slices into a cup of hot water or adding it to green tea.
6. **Green Tea:** If you don't like it, mix it with your Lipton! You will still get its wonderful anti-inflammatory effects. It may reduce the risk of heart disease and cancer.
7. **Tumeric:** This spice is found in many curry spice blends. We also have an excellent pain-relieving supplement with turmeric in it called Pain-Rx. Go to http://www.bellybusterbabe.blogspot.com for a great chicken curry recipe.
8. **Greens:** Fill salads with dark-green lettuce, spinach, and kale.
9. **Cruciferous vegetables:** Broccoli, cauliflower, and brussels sprouts provide another ingredient, sulfur, which helps the body make its own high-powered antioxidants.
10. **Olive oil:** It's a great source of oleic acid, which helps lower blood sugar and is considered an anti-inflammatory oil.

NOTES:_____

_____

_____

On a scale of one to ten, how important is drinking alcohol to you?

_____

5 WHAT IS THE GLYCEMIC INDEX?

Glycemic index (GI) is a measurement of the how carbohydrates in foods affect your blood sugar. It can be used as a tool to help you in losing weight. It works like this: Pure glucose is assigned the value of 100, and other foods are rated relative to glucose by how much they affect blood sugar about two hours after eating.

Foods with a low index typically break down slowly and don't cause drastic fluctuations in blood sugar. Foods with a high index typically do. For instance, broccoli has an index of 10, while cornflakes have an index of 92. Originally, the index was developed to help diabetics control their blood sugar, but the numbers also help people losing weight as well. When the glycemic index is high, you get hungrier as your blood sugar falls. The more your blood sugar falls when it is not under control, the more ravenous you are. If you can keep your blood sugar more stable, your cravings aren't as strong. The index is also helpful for losing weight when you suffer from hypoglycemia (low blood sugar).

Type 2 diabetes, as well as various cancers and cardiovascular disease, are all highly correlated with high index diets. There is abundant research that shows that reducing the overall glycemic index also reduces the risks of those problems.

The index includes mainly carbohydrate foods because protein and fat don't have much immediate effect on blood sugar. Carbohydrates are mostly vegetables, fruits, and starches, like breads and pastas. Proteins are mostly meats, eggs, and nut butters. (We will talk more about healthy and unhealthy fats later, but they are not on the index.) On the Belly Buster Diet, we find the index more helpful than counting calories or grams of fat. We watch whether the foods we're eating have a low, medium, or high index, not the individual index numbers. This can be helpful on any diet in determining how certain foods affects your blood sugar.

As with any rule, there are exceptions. For instance, watermelon has a pretty high glycemic index, about 75, which is even higher than table sugar. Does that make it bad for you? No. In spite of its high index, watermelon actually has a pretty low glycemic load. The glycemic load is a measure based on the amount of a food you'd actually consume (a serving), not just a uniform quantity used in testing for all foods, as with the index.

The glycemic load of a food can be determined using the glycemic index number for a food divided by 100 and multiplied by the number of carbohydrates you'd eat in a reasonable serving of that particular food. With most foods, low index is consistent with low load, but there are the quirky exceptions. Of course, to find them, you'd be back to doing a bunch of math again, and that's just not the way people normally eat.

That's why we encourage dieters to avoid getting caught up in the numbers game and look more generally at the foods in the index, leaning toward those at the low end. Anything over 70 is considered high index, 55 through 69 is medium, and below 55 are foods with a low glycemic index.

Also, look what's in those groups: high index foods include most breakfast cereals, white breads and other processed baked goods, most potatoes, ice cream, candies, and table sugar. Lower index foods include cherries, grapefruit, broccoli, legumes like lentils and beans, most whole grains, and most dairy foods. But if your plan excludes a food, go by what is on your plan, not what is on the index list.

TIP: Fruits tend to have a high glycemic index, so I recommend that people take their fruit with a meal or with a protein, like cottage cheese or regular cheese, that's on their plan. Fruit sugar is released in the bloodstream more slowly when taken with a source of protein. If you snack on a half of an apple, for instance, eat a piece of cheese with it; or if you eat watermelon, eat it with a meal, rather than as an in-between snack.

We like to encourage clients to think of glycemic index and glycemic load as just two more tools that can be helpful in developing healthier dietary habits. You still will need to read labels and watch for fat, sodium, and carb content.

The site "Same Carbohydrate, Different Glycemic Load" (static.diabetesselfmanagement.com/pdfs/DSM032_044.pdf) shows the glycemic load for a variety of the same portions of different foods. The chart below is a summary list common foods and their GI averages. If you want a more complete list, this printable glycemic index chart is another handy resource:

(http://www.health.harvard.edu/newsweek/Glycemic_index_and_glycemic_load_for_100_foods.htm)

Low GI= Under 55
Medium GI = 56 -69
High GI = Greater than 70

Food Categories	Glycemic Index Average (GI)
Apples	Low
Beans	Low
Vegetables	Low
Dairy	Low
Oatmeal and Other Oats	Low
Sweet Potatoes	Low to Medium
Meats and Proteins	None
Legumes	Low
Cereals Very Low in Sugar	Low to Medium
Beverages	
Beer	Medium
Coffee	No effect
Gatorade and Other Sports Drinks	High
Breads	
White Bread	High
Pumpernickel Bread	Low
Rye Bread	High
Flaxseed	Low
Oat Bran	Low
Pita Bread	Medium

Wonder White Bread	High
Whole Wheat Tortillas	Medium
Sourdough	Low
Breakfast Cereals	
All Bran	Low
Bran Flakes	High
Coco Pops	High
Froot Loops	Medium
Frosted Flakes or Special K	Medium
Muesli	Low
Nutri-Grain	Medium
Instant Oatmeal	High
Steel Cut Oats	Low
Puffed Rice	High
Rice Krispies	High
Granola with Dried Fruit or Nuts	High
Muffins and Cakes	
Angel Food Cake	Medium
Banana Bread	Low
Blueberry Muffin	Medium
Carrot Muffin	Medium
Croissant, plain	Medium
Cupcake	High
Pancakes, Premade	Medium to High
Waffles	High
Cereal Grains	
Buckwheat	Low
Millet	High
Quinoa	Low
Bulgur	Low
Polenta	Med
All Dairy Products	**Low**
Fruit, Dried	
Apples	Low
Apricots	Low
Cranberries, Sweetened	Medium
Dates	Low to Medium

Figs	Medium
Prunes	Low
Raisins	Medium
Fruit, Fresh	
Apples	Low
Apricots	Medium
Avocados	Very Low
Banana	Low
Cantaloupe	Medium
Cherries	Medium
Grapefruit	Low
Grapes	Low
Kiwi	Low
Mango	Low
Orange	Low
Papaya	Medium
Peach	Low
Pear	Low
Pineapple	Medium
Strawberries	Low
Watermelon	High
Meat	
Bacon	None
Beef, Lean	None
Calamari	None
All Fish	None
Chicken Nuggets, Breaded	Low
Seafood	None
Fish Sticks	None
Ham	None
Lamb	None
Lobster	None
Turkey	None
Tuna	None
Sushi	Low
Pastas	
Fettuccine Egg Noodles, Cooked	Low
Gnocchi, Cooked	Medium
Instant Noodles (i.e. Ramen Noodles)	Medium
Linguine	Low

Macaroni and Cheese	Medium
Rice	
Basmati Rice	Medium
Brown Rice	Medium
Instant Rice	High
Jasmine Rice	High
Long Grain Rice	Low
Wild Rice	Medium
Candy	
Jelly Beans	High
Licorice, Soft	High
Life Savers	High
Caramel Corn	High
Dark Chocolate	Low
Spreads	
Honey	Low
Agave	Low
Jam (100 percent fruit)	Low
Nutella, Hazelnut Spread, Peanut Butter	Medium
Vegetables	
Corn	High
Beets, Red, Canned	Medium
Broad Beans (Fava)	High
Carrots, Cooked	Low to Medium
Parsnips	High
Potato	High
Most all other Vegetables	Low

NOTES:_____

_____

_____

_____

_____

_____

_____

6 DIET-FRIENDLY SUBSTITUTIONS

Many of the foods we eat on a normal diet slow us down when we are on a weight loss plan. Here are some ideas for substitutions.

Substitutions for Fried Foods

Fried foods should not be a major part of your diet for many reasons, but mainly because foods cooked in this manner are usually high in saturated fat and contain too much sodium. You are at greater risk for high cholesterol and heart disease when you eat a diet that frequently includes them because of the high fat content. Sometimes fried foods and baked goods are also full of preservatives and dyes and other additives that are not good for your health, not to mention full of added calories.

As a researcher, I have gotten a lot of calls about fried foods and cancer because of a chemical called acrylamide that forms if you fry, bake, or roast foods at high temperatures. Some people have used acrylamide as a reason to go to a totally raw diet, but not one single study has shown that acrylamide in the foods we eat is linked with an increased risk of cancer. Many occupational and environmental exposures can occur to cause people to have a much higher level of acrylamide in their bodies than eating fried food. Regardless of this, fried potatoes and baked snacks should not be a major part of our diet for many other reasons. Fried foods are fine for an occasional treat when you are at a maintenance weight, but when you're in weight loss mode, search out substitute recipes for things that taste just as good, but are not fried, broiled, or processed.

For example, a fried chicken breast has 80 percent more calories and four times the fat of a skinless, grilled, or baked chicken breast. A grilled or baked one has no carbohydrates, but if you add flour or a batter to the skin, you also add carbs.

I use cooking sprays like Pam to coat meats and vegetables with either panko crumbs or, my favorite, a mixture of crushed Melba toast and herbs (usually I just mix it with a packet of our dry chicken soup mix from the Before and After Weight Loss Clinic, but you can use Mrs. Dash and get a similar taste.) If you season your chicken with a mixture of a little Badia Sazon Tropical (the one without monosodium glutamate [MSG]), and a smidgeon of McCormick Extra Spicy with a couple of tablespoons of Bisquick or gluten-free baking mix, it tastes just like KFC when you bake it!

Here are some recipes for baked instead of fried substitutions. I promise you these zucchini fries have more flavor than any french fry you ever put in your mouth!

Zucchini Fries (for those dieting)
2 medium zucchini, peeled and cut like fries
1 egg, well-beaten or equivalent Egg Beaters
20 pieces Melba toast, crushed in blender
1/4 cup Parmesan cheese
1 packet low-sodium dry soup mix (If you cannot find protein soup like ours, use herbs like Mrs. Dash)

Dip the zucchini sticks in the egg and then in the Melba toast, herb, and soup mixture until coated. Cover the toaster oven tray with foil and bake in toaster at 350 degrees for 25 to 30 min. or until golden brown. Serves 4. Great with grilled hamburger patties.

Jo Jo's Baked Potato "Fries" (for those maintaining)
4 medium white potatoes, diced
1/4 cup flour or cornmeal (optional)
1/4 cup Parmesan cheese
1 tablespoon Mrs. Dash
1 teaspoon rosemary or oregano

½ teaspoon black pepper
cooking spray

Spray a Pyrex dish with cooking spray. Spray diced potatoes with it, too, so that herbs will stick well. Mix herbs and flour or meal together. Dredge the potatoes in the mixture and then place in the dish. Bake at 375 degrees for 35 to 40 minutes. Serves 4.

<u>Baked Okra</u>

If you miss fried okra, try baking it! I bake it and then add it to the above potato recipe without the cheese. Okra is very low in calories: 1 cup has just 38 calories, less than 8 grams of carbohydrates, and less than 1 gram of fat. When you bake it, and spray a little cooking spray on it, amazingly the okra tastes fried.

Substitutes for Eggs—or Not?

Eggs aren't just for Easter! Research now shows that eggs eaten at the start of the day can reduce daily calorie intake, prevent snacking between meals, and keep you satisfied on those busy days when mealtime is delayed. Research also suggests that high-quality protein foods such as lean meat and eggs can keep your appetite satisfied longer, aid in your weight loss, and help preserve your lean muscle mass.

One egg provides 6 grams of protein, or 12 percent of the Recommended Daily Value. Eggs provide perhaps the highest quality protein found in any food because they contain all of the essential amino acids our bodies need. Many people think the egg white has all the protein, but it is actually the yolk that provides nearly half of it. The yolk is also where most of the cholesterol is found, so you can eat egg whites or Egg Beaters if you prefer. You don't have to use egg whites to lower your cholesterol, though, because the guidelines have changed. The old guidelines said to consume no more than one real egg per day if you have high cholesterol or are on cholesterol medication, and no more than two if you have normal cholesterol. Now research shows that blood cholesterol does not increase with the dietary intake of foods with cholesterol; in fact, these foods help your body produce less of its own. The current recommendation of up to three eggs per day goes for everyone!

Eating eggs for breakfast as part of a reduced-calorie diet helped overweight people on our diet at Before and After Weight Loss Clinics in Florida lose 65 percent more weight and lower their Body Mass Index (BMI) by 61 percent more than dieters who ate another nationally recognized diet with the same number of calories but had a bagel-based, carb-laden breakfast. Our clients who ate eggs for breakfast also boasted an amazing 85 percent greater reduction in waist circumference and also much greater improvements in their energy levels than their counterparts on the bagel breakfast. Our results were almost identical to those from the research in a similar study at Louisiana State University. At LSU they also found that the people who ate the eggs for breakfast consumed an average of 330 fewer calories throughout the day than adults who ate a bagel-based breakfast.

One of my clients brought me this delicious zucchini frittata recipe for breakfast. Granted, on the Belly Buster Diet, we are supposed to have scallions (green onions) rather than sweet onions—they call them sweet because they have more sugar in them—so you can use scallions instead if you wish. During your maintenance phase you could add a couple of tablespoons of low-fat Bisquick to it to make it more like a quiche. Try it with different cheeses, but Gruyere or Swiss cheese are my favorites.

Asparagus or Zucchini Frittata Recipe
2 teaspoons canola oil
1/2 small onion, thinly sliced
1/2 teaspoon salt
1 pound asparagus spears, tough ends snapped off, cut diagonally into 1-inch lengths;
or 1/2 cup peeled and diced zucchini
4 large eggs, lightly beaten (or Egg Beaters)
1 cup shredded Gruyere or Swiss cheese

Heat oil in a 10-inch ovenproof frying pan over medium high heat. Add onions and salt and cook, stirring occasionally, until onions are softened. Add asparagus; reduce heat to low, and cook covered until the asparagus are barely tender; about 8 minutes. Pour in eggs and cook until almost set, but runny on top. While cooking, preheat oven broiler. Sprinkle cheese over eggs and put in oven to broil until cheese is melted and browned. Remove and cut into wedges on serving plate. Serves 4.

TIPS: Of course, how you prepare your eggs counts! A large egg has only 1.5 grams of saturated fat and about 70 calories. However, a bacon, egg & cheese biscuit sandwich from McDonald's has 12 grams of saturated fat (59 percent of the daily value for someone eating a 2,000 calorie diet) and 420 calories, not to mention 1,130 milligrams of sodium. I microwave mine or boil them. Boiled eggs also make a great snack between meals. Keep boiled eggs or deviled eggs in the refrigerator, and go light on the salt, mayo, and relish.

Substitutes for Pastas

One cup of regular egg noodles has about 40 grams of carbohydrates. On most diets, including ours at Before and After Weight Loss Clinics, that is way too many carbohydrates in a serving. The good news is that we now have oodles of noodle alternatives!

My favorite alternative to pasta is spaghetti squash, a yellow football-shaped squash whose strands can be scraped from the center. The strands look just like spaghetti noodles. The squash can be purchased just about year-round and cooks in just 12 minutes in the microwave. But if you want something that tastes more like Italian pasta or Japanese noodles, I recommend two other alternatives: Miracle Noodles, which you can get at a health food store or on the internet, or Shirataki noodles, which you can purchase at your local grocer.

Miracle Noodles contain no gluten, have zero net carbs, no fat, no calories, and are made of a water-soluble natural fiber called glucomannan. The glucomannan in Miracle Noodles helps slow the absorption of glucose, which then slows the release of insulin from the pancreas, thus keeping blood glucose levels more normal after eating a meal. For this reason, it is a great product for people with Type 2 diabetes. These noodles don't have a lot of taste and take on the taste of whatever you are mixing with it. With all the fiber, you will *not* have constipation once you eat them!

Shirataki noodles are the same, but with a little tofu added for texture. They are found in the vegetarian section of your grocer and smell like seaweed when you open the bag. But don't throw them out! Just dump them in a colander and rinse them with the sprayer ten times—no really, ten times! Then pat the noodles dry with a paper towel and cut them into smaller pieces with kitchen scissors. Place them on a plate and put in the microwave for one minute and the smell disappears. They are then ready to eat and taste just like pasta! Shirataki comes in spaghetti noodles and several thicker noodles, like fettuccini. Half the bag is a serving with only 20 calories and 3 grams of carbohydrates!

You can turn lots of dishes that are traditionally high carb into low-carb dishes with these noodles: traditional spaghetti with low-carb Classico tomato sauce or Walden Farms alfredo sauce over them, like chicken noodle soup, and turkey tetrazzini, to name a few. Check out our clinics' recipe blog for other recipes at www.bellybusterbabe.blogspot.com. Wait to use the low-carb noodles like Barilla when you are ready to maintain your weight.

Here is one of my favorites that includes a gravy recipe you can use in other recipes:

Swedish Meatballs Over Shirataki Fettuccine
This recipe can be made with dry soup or diet protein soup powder.
Meatballs:
1 pound of ground beef, chicken, or turkey
1 dry packet of Before and After chicken soup protein powder with herb seasonings
1 egg

Gravy:
1 small carton of Friendship Dairies no-salt cottage cheese
1 packet of Before and After beef soup protein powder
4 ounces water
8 ounces mushrooms
1 teaspoon Worcestershire sauce or Kitchen Bouquet
1 teaspoon onion powder
pepper, garlic powder, and nutmeg to taste
spaghetti squash or Shirataki fettuccini or noodles

Make meatballs with the first three ingredients. (Use crushed Melba toast if you don't have our soup.) Bake at 350 degrees on a cookie sheet sprayed with oil for 30 minutes. Blend water, soup mix, sauce, and cottage cheese in blender until smooth. Pour this mixture over the other ingredients and the meatballs in a skillet and bring to a boil. Cook down and serve over noodles. Freezes well.

Substitutions for Diet Sodas

Water. That's it. There are no other substitutions.

The average American drinks more than forty gallons of soda per year. Since 1978, shortly before Diet Coke was invented, soda consumption has tripled for boys and doubled for girls. It's like we thought taking out the sugar made it really healthy to drink! We have all heard how horrible diet soda is for your body, but how many of us really pay attention to any of that when we want to lose weight? But do you really know the facts behind the rumors? I love my Diet Coke, and every time I pick the habit back up, I have a hard time breaking it. Last time, I swore Coca-Cola must have started putting cocaine in it again because I was surely addicted! So, I set out to do some research to find out why my body craves this drink so much that it seems to sabotage my dieting efforts—and boy, did I find out plenty! And, you should know about this, too.

1) Diet soda triggers sweet receptors on the tongue, but may or may not trigger your insulin. If it doesn't, you never feel full, and it causes you to actually crave more food and perhaps eat more sugary or high-carb foods to get a fix. If it does, the insulin will not be used because there is no glucose available, and you will become insulin resistant over the long haul.

2) Studies from the University of Minnesota showed that just one diet soda a day is linked to a 34 percent higher risk of metabolic syndrome, a disorder with a cluster of symptoms that, combined, slows down metabolism and therefore slows weight loss. Having three of these symptoms is considered metabolic syndrome:
   - belly fat
   - high fasting glucose
   - high triglycerides
   - elevated blood pressure
   - low HDL (good) cholesterol

3) Studies at the University of Texas showed that drinking two or more cans of diet soda a day could increase your

weight by up to 500 percent. The study said that the more diet soda you drink, the greater your risk of becoming or remaining overweight. In part, it could be the artificial sweeteners, and alternatively, the caramel coloring that inhibits proper protein metabolism in the liver.

4) A study at Purdue University concerning artificial sweeteners in diet sodas proved that they disrupt your body's natural ability to regulate calorie intake, making you crave more food. One diet soda a day increased the likelihood of diabetes by 36 percent and Type 2 diabetes by 67 percent. The study also showed a 30 percent increase in depression among the participants who drank diet soda. At the University of Sheffield in the United Kingdom, Dr. Peter Piper found that diet sodas contain something that regular sodas don't: mold inhibitors. Potassium benzoate is a preservative, and it severely damages the DNA in your mitochondria, making them totally inactive. If your mitochondria are inactive, then they are not producing energy and your metabolism is not at full throttle.

If you need more than weight management to motivate you not to drink diet sodas, there are a few other healthful hints. Researchers found that diet soda is associated with a twofold risk for kidney problems in those that just drank two or more per day. Adults who drink three or more sodas per day have far greater tooth decay, more missing teeth, and more fillings. Also, soda cans are lined with the endocrine disruptor bisphenol A (BPA), which has been linked to everything from heart disease to obesity to reproductive problems.

Get an insulated water bottle and keep ice and water in it. Take it everywhere. Try drinking no diet soda and drinking lots of water this month. I guarantee you that you will start craving the water and won't miss the bubbly.

Substitute Organic Soy Milk for Dairy Milk

I grew up on a dairy farm and drank milk with cream in it until I went to college. The worst part of freshman year was getting used to drinking that diluted milk that my parents told me was pasteurized and homogenized and quite different than the rich dairy milk I loved so much. However, it was not long after I graduated from college that my dad had a heart attack in his mid-fifties, and he became as much of a health food fanatic as I am. And what did he do about that cow's milk? Although he had been in the dairy industry for years, he switched to soy milk! (I was shocked, but you should also know that he grew soybeans as well as raising cattle.)

Soy milk is great for heart patients and great for losing weight because it is low in fat, low in calories if you drink plain or unsweetened, and has a lower glycemic index than dairy milk, almond milk, or rice milk. The plain soy milk only has 4 grams of carbs in a half-cup to the 8 grams in a half-cup of skim milk, and 45 calories versus the 60 in skim milk. Soy milk also has much less saturated fat. Many people are lactose intolerant and don't know it until they switch to soy milk. When they don't have the constant bloating and flatulence any longer, they figure it out. What a nice surprise!

Despite all these great facts, many myths have been spread about soy milk that are simply untrue—and unfortunately, sometimes even doctors inadvertently repeat them. For instance, some will tell you if you have cancer or thyroid disease, you cannot drink any amount of soy milk. Let's set the record straight. I got this request via email recently, and I have been getting this question for years in my clinics since whole soy foods are on our menus: "My oncologist asked me not to have soy, saying it produces estrogen and would stimulate cancer growth. In all of the information I have read, I cannot find anything that supports this. On the contrary, I have found that it may actually reduce breast cancer risk. Is it safe for a person with a history of breast cancer to eat soy foods or not?"

As with most confusing nutrition topics, there is a grain of truth to the concept that soy foods are related to estrogen. However, the concept that soy foods produce estrogen, and therefore are unsafe for women with a history of breast cancer, is very misleading. I also hear it in relation to people with thyroid disease. If you do not take it *with* your thyroid medication and instead wait the same length of time you wait for anything else with calcium in it, you can drink soy *in moderation* with no problem.

Researchers have noted that women who traditionally consume soy food as part of a normal diet, such as Japanese women, have much lower breast cancer rates as compared to women who do not eat soy foods regularly. The results of these studies *may or may not* apply to women in other countries besides Japan. It is important to note that there are many differences in diet and lifestyle between Japanese and non-Japanese women. For example, Japanese women often are thinner, they may exercise more, they may have other differences in their diet, and they may have different patterns of childbearing as compared to non-Japanese women. Furthermore, Japanese women who eat soy foods may have higher quality diets overall; they may eat more fruits and vegetables, and they may eat less total fat. Any of these factors may play a role in the differences in breast cancer risk between Japanese and non-Japanese women.

A large portion of research about women who eat soy foods in adulthood supports that it is safe and may reduce risk of breast cancer. Soy foods contain dozens of different nutrients that appear to have many important functions in our bodies. They protect cells from damage, encourage damaged cells to die (rather than to keep multiplying), provide vital nutrients that control normal cell growth, and enhance cell-to-cell communication.

However, we cannot assume that simply adding soy foods to the diet automatically will reduce the risk of breast cancer.

The idea that soy foods are related to human estrogen comes from the fact that these foods do contain a group of nutrients that are known as phytoestrogens or plant estrogens. This term caught on because soy foods do contain some nutrients that look chemically similar to some of the estrogens that occur naturally in the human body. Unfortunately, the term "phytoestrogen" caught on in the media. Many people, including health care providers, focus on that one aspect of this very complex food. In truth, soy foods appear to have many cancer fighting abilities, many of which do not have anything to do with any type of so-called estrogen activity. However, because the popular literature focuses only on the phytoestrogen aspects of soy foods, many people have the mistaken idea that soy literally contains or makes estrogen. This is not true. However, in defense of health care providers, it is important to remember that it is very difficult to keep up on all of the research literature on any one topic. Thousands of studies are published every year just on cancer and nutrition alone.

Many studies have been done about soy and you can read more about them online.(Check out http://www.cancer.gov, www.touchedbycancer.org/surviorship/cancer-and-nutrtion, etc.)

and In the meantime, think of estrogen as a key that fits in a lock in a cell and unlocks cancer should you be prone to it; think of a phytoestrogen as key that fits the keyhole, but cannot turn the lock and blocks the estrogen from the cell. I firmly believe that soy protects you from cancer, and that is why I drink organic soy milk and eat whole soy foods.

Whole organic soy foods, not processed, are the key. I believe that *whole soy foods* (tofu, tempeh, miso, soy milk) can and should be included in the diet of women with a history of breast cancer. Soy foods should be one part, but not the whole focus of a healthy, cancer-fighting diet. No one, especially not women with a history of breast cancer, should consume highly processed soy foods (soy supplements, soy hot dogs, soy chips, soy fortified cereals, etc.). These foods do not contain the same balance of healthy nutrients as whole soy food, such as tofu, tempeh, or miso. Plus, they often contain many unhealthy ingredients such as preservatives, colorings, and sodium.

Soy milk smoothies have been part of my diet for breakfast and snacks and have not caused a change in my thyroid despite being on medication, and I still test negative for any form of cancer. Here is one of my favorite soy smoothie recipes that you can use with a variety of fruits.

Berry Soy Smoothie
½ cup plain organic soy milk
1 packet Before and After strawberry protein gelatin
or 1 packet Knox gelatin
¼ cup blueberries, frozen
5 strawberries, frozen
½ cup ice

Blend first two ingredients in blender then add the other three. Sweeten with liquid Stevia drops. Makes one serving. (Stevia and protein are sold at the Before and After clinic.) You can vary this by adding different frozen fruits: pineapple, peaches, mango, and cherries. You can also add canned pumpkin or PB2. If you are maintaining your weight, add bananas, pears, or peanut butter. For more recipes, see our blog at www.bellybusterbabe.blogspot.com.

If you are allergic to soy, try almond milk. If you are allergic to both soy and nuts, stick with 1 percent or skim milk. Hood makes low-carb milk. Just be aware of carbs and glycemic index when choosing what is best and consider whether your diet is calorie-, fat-, or carb-restrictive or if certain foods are strictly forbidden.

TIP: Did you know that some of the latest research the American Heart Association has released says that having three servings of different-colored berries per week leads to a 75 percent lower chance of having a heart attack? Soy shakes are a great way to get them in and lose weight at the same time!

Substitutions for Bread
Some diets allow some grains and forbid others, so be sure that whatever is suggested here goes along with the weight loss plan you are following. If you are allergic to wheat like I am, you may need to have your counselor come up with other grains or starch sources to balance your diet, but you should not totally leave off a source of starch or you will become constipated. I recommend that you take at least one psyllium capsule per day to ensure proper fiber intake if you are following a low-fat, low-carb, high-protein plan like the Belly Buster Diet. We carry psyllium (the "p" is silent) on our website and in our clinics. If you are chronically constipated, take Miralax from the pharmacy.

TIP: If you are allergic to wheat, you can take a product called GlutenEase that has enzymes to help you digest wheat if you forget and eat wheat anyway. It has been a lifesaver for me, as I had no idea why I was up all night with my ears and throat itching.

If you are on a diet that allows low-carb bread, try five rounds of Melba toast or 8 Crunchmaster gluten-free crackers (from Sam's Club), Nature's Own 40-calorie bread, or Sara Lee 45-calorie bread. Limit low-carb tortillas to just three per week because of the extra fat and sodium, and use the smaller size ones (about the size of a small bread plate), which have 3 grams of net carbohydrates and only 50 calories each. My favorite brand is La Tortilla Factory, but there are many others. La Tortilla Factory also makes pita pockets that are low-carb. These freeze well, so if you only do one or two a week, you won't have to throw away the rest of the bag. You can substitute bib lettuce and make lettuce "tortillas" instead.

Here are a dozen ideas for quick low-carb meals or snacks using low-carb pitas or tortillas:

Quesadillas: Put cheese between two tortillas—have half with lettuce wraps.

Chicken fajita: Use chicken strips, peppers, and onion with Tajin spice. (See recipe below.)

Chicken salad wrap: Go light on the mayo by using Hellmann's Dijonnaise and/or Walden Farms mayonnaise mixed with lite mayonnaise.

Shrimp stir-fry wrap: Combine shrimp with mixed veggies, asparagus, and a dash of Braggs Amino Acids (a replacement sauce for soy sauce).

Breakfast burrito: Add eggs and peppers with salsa.

Beef Asian wrap: Mix beef strips with teriyaki sauce or Thick N Spicy Walden Farms Barbeque Sauce. Wrap in bibb lettuce. You can use beef or chicken.

Pizza: Coat low-carb tortilla with Classico Florentine tomato sauce and veggies, low-fat meat, and cheese. Hormel makes a pepperoni that is 70 percent fat-free that you can use sparingly.

Pita chips and salsa: Toast a whole tortilla and then slice with pizza cutter into eight pieces.

Cinnamon chips: Bake coated with Promise and sprinkle with cinnamon and ¼ teaspoon sugar. Cut into eighths with a pizza cutter.

Beef taco: Combine ground beef and chili powder—don't use packaged (high sodium).

Fish taco: Combine tilapia and broccoli slaw and homemade low-fat tartar sauce.

Fluffer Nutter: Mix PB2 with Walden Farms marshmallow dip and spread on tortilla—oh my goodness! (Before and After Weight Loss Clinics carries both of these products.)

Here is an easy recipe for fajitas that you can use with beef or chicken.

Chicken Fajitas
8 ounces boneless chicken breast strips
2 large bib lettuce leaves, or 2 low-carb tortillas
½ green pepper, in slices

¼ cup onions or scallions
1 teaspoon Mrs. Dash Extra Spicy Seasoning Blend
1 ounce water
½ small tomato, diced
2 tablespoons salsa
1 tablespoon plain non-fat yogurt

Stir-fry pepper, onions, chicken, and seasonings in the water. Place half the mixture on each lettuce leaf or tortilla. Top with tomato, salsa, and yogurt. Carefully roll lettuce or tortilla around mixture like a burrito.

Substitutions for Desserts

Aaahhh! I saved the best for last! We all like a treat or two, even on a diet, but it does not have to be after *every* meal. Decide on your three favorite desserts and learn to make those three in a more dietetic way. Then have them on special occasions. My favorites are cheesecake, tiramisu, and ice cream. I am able to make all of them with our protein supplements and each one is so simple.

For the cheesecakes, I have a recipe for each month. I use different flavorings, depending on the month. That keeps it fresh with something to look forward to without getting bored. I will give you the list of ideas for that, but first here is the basic recipe for an Unbelievable Cheesecake.

Unbelievable Cheesecake

6 eggs (or Egg Beaters equivalent)
1 tablespoon lemon juice
1 package vanilla crème pudding protein supplement (or 2 scoops protein powder)
1 package lemon protein supplement (or 2 scoops lemon or strawberry protein)
1 packet Knox gelatin
24 ounces 1% low-fat cottage cheese
fresh fruit
Cool Whip

Blend all ingredients in a blender. Spray a deep 8x8 pan; pour in batter. Bake for 30 min—*no longer*—at 350 degrees. Turn off oven and leave cheesecake in oven *with door open* for 1 hour. Chill overnight. Serve with fruit and Cool Whip. **TIP:** The Knox gelatin keeps it from getting watery in the refrigerator. Serves 6.

Here is an idea for a cheesecake every month:

January: Comstock light cherry pie filling on top.

February: Strawberry gelatin and strawberries.

March: Lime gelatin and pineapple for St Patrick's Day.

April: Raspberry gelatin with raspberries on top.

May: Pineapple drink and pudding mix with ½ cup drained pineapple throughout or on bottom for pineapple upside-down cake.

June: Piña colada cheesecake with 2/3 cup crushed pineapple (drained), and Watkins coconut and banana flavorings.

July: The basic recipe topped with blueberries for the season.

August: Double chocolate decadence made with Before and After chocolate pudding and Walden Farms chocolate syrup.

September: Chocolate amaretto made with one packet of Before and After amaretto hot cocoa.

October: Pumpkin (1/2 can) with pineapple on top.

November: Pumpkin (1/2 can) with cinnamon for Thanksgiving.

December: Mint cocoa mix throughout with a few crushed peppermints on top.

Dream up a flavor of your own:

_____

_____

_____

_____

NOTES and other favorite substitutions or recipes from the

website:_____

_____

_____

_____

_____

_____

_____

_____

_____

_____

_____

_____

_____

_____

_____

_____

_____

_____

_____

7 CAN FATS MAKE YOU FAT?

Yes, fat makes you fat! But, ironically, small quantities of *good* fats must be present in order for you to lose weight. Overindulging in foods that have a lot of the wrong fat can lead to weight gain; but to be healthy, a diet should include some good fat. Anything with trans fats, however, should be avoided, like fried food, ice cream, coffee creamers, popcorn, and margarine. There are plenty of great, healthy fats that can and should be incorporated into your diet. Avocados, nuts (not honey roasted), and olive oil are three great sources of fat that you can incorporate into your diet and still lose weight. Check to see what each phase of your diet allows; some diets allow different fats in different phases of their plans.

One way to increase weight loss with small amounts of these good oils is to eat foods with conjugated linoleic acid (CLA) in them. Canola oil, or even better, safflower oil, are the preferred oils while dieting because they both have a huge amount of CLA. I like the nutty taste of the safflower oil, but it does go rancid faster. (Olive oil does not have very much CLA in it, but you can go back to it when you reach your maintenance weight. CLA helps you lose fat faster but not necessarily to lose weight faster. It is a key ingredient in our EFA (Essential Fatty Acid) capsules and also has these other benefits:

75

- **CLA lowers cholesterol and triglycerides.** Take it with cinnamon to see dramatic results.
- **It increases metabolic rate.** This is a benefit, especially for thyroid patients.
- **CLA decreases abdominal fat.** Adrenal imbalances and hormonal shifts are common in thyroid patients and other overweight patients. They cause rapid accumulation of abdominal fat.
- **It enhances muscle growth.** Muscle burns fat, which also contributes to increased metabolism.
- **CLA lowers insulin resistance.** Lowering insulin can also help prevent adult-onset diabetes and make it easier to control weight.
- **It reduces food-induced allergic reactions.** Since food allergies may be at play when weight loss becomes difficult, this can be of help to thyroid patients.
- **CLA enhances the immune system.** Since most cases of thyroid disease are autoimmune in nature, enhancing the immune system's ability to function properly may help.

TIP: I strongly recommend that no matter what weight loss plan you follow, you take either EFA, CLA, or flaxseed oil capsules. Any one of those will enhance your fat loss.

What About Peanut Butter?
In just 2 tablespoons, peanut butter has about 16 grams fat, 8 grams of carbohydrates, and 190 calories. Now if you add bread or crackers or jelly, your diet is screwed! Never fear; there is a solution! First, do not bring Jif home from the grocer with you—or any food that you have no control over, for that matter. Second, purchase some PB2, powdered peanut butter. It is the powdery by-product of squeezing the oil out of peanuts. To reconstitute it, add two tablespoons of PB2 powder to one tablespoon of water. You can put it on apples or Melba toast or in puddings and shakes. PB2 does not spread well unless you add Walden Farms marshmallow, chocolate, or caramel dip to it. Then it is sweeter and glides just fine. And you cut the fat by a whooping 85 percent, and it only has 45 calories, 5 grams of carbohydrates, and 5 grams of protein.

My favorite thing to do with PB2 is put it in Before and After double chocolate pudding protein mix and made a milkshake with it. This incredible smoothie tastes like you are drinking a Snickers bar! Most of these ingredients can be found on our website at www.bestdietsource.com.

Chocolate Caramel Peanut Butter Milkshake
1/2 cup soy milk (or Hood's Calorie Countdown dairy beverage (a low-carb diary milk) if allergic to soy or almond milk)

8 ounces water

2 heaping teaspoons PB2

1 packet of Before and After chocolate drink or a scoop of protein powder

1 heaping tablespoon Walden Farms caramel dip

1 packet sweetener *or* 3 drops Stevia if desired

1 cup of ice

Blend all ingredients in a blender with a good ice crusher setting. Sweeten to taste.

PB2 and Jelly Sandwich
1 slice 40- or 45-calorie bread (or gluten-free bread, if that is what your menu calls for)

2 tablespoons PB2, prepared according to package directions

1 teaspoon Walden Farms marshmallow dip

1 tablespoon sugar-free apricot preserves or blackberry jelly

Mix the PB2 and marshmallow dip together to give it a sweeter taste and help it glide on the bread. After spreading it on the bread (toasted or untoasted), spread the jelly. Eat open-faced.

What About Fats and Carbs in the Crock-Pot?
Many people put their Crock-Pots in the closet when they are dieting because so many of the recipes for Crock-Pots have rich gravies with high quantities of unhealthy fat. Never fear! With a few belly bustin' tips, your Crock-Pot can be back in service with low-carb, low-fat recipes that get you skinny in no time flat! They are wonderful when you work long hours.

To get ready to use your crock, make a list of what meats your family likes. My list consisted of chicken (breasts and whole), turkey (breast), beef (stew, rump roast, and chuck roast), and pork (chops and shoulder). Then make a list of what low-carb and low-fat sauces your family likes. Mine are chicken and beef broth, Walden Farms barbeque sauce and honey Dijon dressing, Classico tomato sauces, Ro*Tel tomatoes, and Del Monte diced tomatoes. From these meats and sauces, you can come up with all sorts of combinations. If you are not sure what spices to add, just add Mrs. Dash—she goes with everything and makes everything tastes great!

You can also do vegetables in the Crock-Pot too. One of my favorites is stuffed green peppers. Put low-sodium beef broth in the bottom of the crock—about an inch deep. Stuff the peppers with 3 tablespoons of ground beef and 1 tablespoon each of cottage cheese, Swiss cheese, oatmeal, and dried apples coated with cinnamon. If you don't want to use oatmeal and apples, try quartering button mushrooms and using 1 tablespoon of Ro*Tel tomatoes instead. Top with a little more cheese and slow-cook for about 4 hours. The texture of the mushrooms makes it taste like there are beans in it, but there are none. My crock will hold five of these.

One of our clients recently reached her goal of losing 100 pounds! She gave us this recipe. It can be modified to taste and can also be used as a marinade and a salad dressing. I added honey Dijon dressing and put it in the Crock-Pot. It can be used on pork as well.

Chicken in Apricot Vinaigrette Glaze (Sweet and Sour Chicken)
½ bottle Walden Farms honey Dijon salad dressing
4 chicken breasts
½ green bell pepper
½ red bell pepper

Base Glaze
¼ cup apple cider
¼ cup sugar-free apricot preserves
1 tablespoon Dijon mustard
3 tablespoon sugar-free pancake syrup

Mix half of the base glaze with a half of a bottle of Walden Farms honey Dijon salad dressing. Put four chicken breasts in the Crock-Pot and slice a half a green pepper and half of a red pepper over them. Pour the Dijon mixture over the chicken and peppers.

Cook in the crock on low for 4 to 5 hours. Heat the remaining base glaze in the microwave and serve over the chicken when done.

One meat I really love in the Crock-Pot is pork. I don't eat ham because the sodium makes me swell, but lean pork chops and pork shoulders do well in a crock and have only about 1 gram of fat and 3 grams of carbohydrates when prepared this way. I recommend that you do not eat ham until maintaining your goal weight and that you never eat cured ham because of the salt and nitrates in it.

Perfect Pulled Pork
1 5-pound pork butt (shoulder)
½ cup water
1 ½ teaspoon smoked paprika
½ teaspoon salt
2 teaspoons pepper
2 teaspoons cayenne

Cook all ingredients in Crock-Pot on high for 4 to 5 hours. Pull meat apart. Serve as is, or sprinkle in a little vinegar or serve with Walden Farms Original or Thick & Spicy Barbeque Sauce. I have added the sauce or vinegar to the crock ahead of time and I have added a Diet Dr. Pepper to the crock before too. Every time, I say it is the best barbeque I have ever had.

What fats do you have a hard time staying away from?

_____

_____

_____

_____

What are good fats you can eat on your diet?

_____

_____

_____

_____

NOTES:_____

8 FOOD ALLERGIES, IRRITABLE BOWEL SYNDROME, AND GLUTEN SENSITIVITY

Food allergies, irritable bowel syndrome (IBS), and gluten sensitivity can all contribute to weight problems because of the inflammation they cause in the body. When you eat a food you are allergic to, your adrenal glands release the hormones cortisol and adrenalin (also called epinephrine) to respond to the allergic reaction. This sets off a chain reaction: These hormones cause a breakdown of stored carbohydrates in the liver called glycogen and increases your blood sugar level, which then stimulates the release of insulin. However, the high cortisol levels direct your cells to stop taking sugar up from the blood, resulting in temporary insulin resistance. So the cells do not take up the glucose just released into the blood, creating an even higher insulin level. The high level of insulin activates the enzyme lipoprotein lipase, which catalyzes the production of fats and promotes the storage fat you eat rather than using it for fuel. The high insulin levels also inhibit the activity of the enzyme triglyceride lipase that breaks down stored fat for use as energy.

Thus, if you have chronically high insulin due to continual inflammation in your gut, you cannot burn your own body fat, and any fat you eat is likely to be stored rather than used for energy. In addition, in the next two hours after a meal, if your insulin level is high, protein and carbohydrates you eat that are in excess of what you burn for fuel are more likely to be converted to and stored as fat as well.

The inflammation from food allergies or from wheat or gluten sensitivity also makes leptin, the master weight control hormone, ineffective. Overweight people usually have very high levels of leptin, but become leptin resistant with repeated flares of inflammation because the C-reactive protein binds to the leptin. If an optimally healthy, normal-weight person overeats, their leptin level rises, which increases their metabolic rate and decreases their appetite. However, that does not happen if you have constant inflammation due to food allergies, irritable bowel, or gluten sensitivity, like celiac disease.

The symptoms of food allergies can be quite varied. I had a severe wheat allergy for years before I figured out what was literally keeping me up all night. After I ate something with wheat in it, I did not have an immediate reaction, but I would be up all night with itching in my ears and throat! I wish I had read somewhere that this meant I was allergic to a food and not to dust mites or to whatever detergent I used for the bed linens.

A wheat allergy should not be confused with gluten intolerance or celiac disease. A food allergy is an overreaction of the immune system to a specific food protein. When the food protein is ingested, it can trigger an allergic reaction that may include a range of symptoms from mild symptoms such as rashes, hives, itching, and swelling to severe symptoms like trouble breathing, wheezing, or loss of consciousness. A food allergy can even be potentially fatal.

Celiac disease, which affects the small intestines, is caused by an abnormal immune reaction to gluten. It is a digestive disease usually diagnosed by a gastroenterologist. When left untreated, it can cause serious complications, including malnutrition and intestinal damage. Individuals with celiac disease must avoid gluten, found in wheat, rye, barley, and sometimes oats.

People who are allergic to wheat often tolerate other grains. However, about 20 percent of children with a wheat allergy are also allergic to other grains. They should be tested to see what else they can and cannot tolerate.

TIP: Did you know that you can lose a significant amount of weight by cutting food allergens from your diet and taking probiotics for a while? If you get rid of the inflammation and balance the bacterial ecosystem in your intestinal tract, you will lose weight much more efficiently. Probiotics are inexpensive and found in most pharmacies and health food stores, as well as on our website.

Another way you can get inflammation in your intestinal system is simply eating the typical American diet of high sugar, high carbs, and high fat. The typical American diet actually fosters the growth of bacteria and yeasts in the gut. They damage the lining and produce toxins that are absorbed into your system. Because of the damage, partially digested food particles can also leak into your bloodstream. Then your immune system reacts to the toxins and foods, producing a firestorm of inflammation. That inflammation then leads to a fatty liver and insulin resistance, which leads to higher levels of insulin in your body. Insulin makes you heavier because it is a fat-storage, disease- and aging-promoting hormone.

Tips For Those with Irritable Bowel Syndrome

Irritable bowel syndrome can be hard to diagnose, and the symptoms can be similar to gluten sensitivity and celiac disease. Often clients come to us with gas, bloating, and stomach discomfort, but have no idea why they have so many different digestive problems. Major Joshua Watson, M.D., who is a gastroenterologist at Dwight D. Eisenhower Army Medical Center in Fort Gordon, Georgia, oversees the medical end of our weight loss business. He urges that someone with these symptoms first be tested for celiac disease, and if the test for celiac is negative, then have your doctor test for gluten sensitivities. It is also possible to be allergic to one grain and not another. For instance, you can be allergic to wheat, but not necessarily allergic to gluten or other grains.

You can do an elimination diet if think you have food allergies or IBS and you are struggling to lose weight. However, you should not do it if you suspect you have celiac disease because the antibodies need to be present when a doctor is testing you and antibodies will not be if you have already eliminated the foods. You should go to a gastroenterologist first and rule that out. Here are a few simple things to try to eliminate food allergens and rebalance your intestinal flora.

1) **Try an elimination diet for 3 weeks.** Cut out the most common food allergens, including gluten, dairy, eggs, corn, yeast, peanuts, and those foods to which you know you are

allergic. Add them back one at a time. I knew within three days that I was severely allergic to wheat—it was undeniably evident. You will be surprised.

2) **Eat a whole-food, plant-based, high-fiber diet.** This is essential to feed the good bacteria in your gut and to provide the nutrients you need to functional optimally during this time.

3) **Take probiotics daily to boost the healthy bacteria in your gut.** Look for those reputable brands, like Before and After or Jarrow, that contain both bifidobacteria and lactobacillus.

Within a very few short weeks—even if you do nothing else—you will see a dramatic difference that comes from healing your gut. Remember, if you want to get rid of that gut, you have to fix your gut.

I recommend these products during your three-week elimination diet:

- Pamela's baking mix (It's gluten-free)
- Crunchmaster crackers (from Sam's Club)
- Before and After probiotics (available at any of our clinics)
- Before and After Protein weight loss shakes (available at any of our clinics)

In 2011, researchers first hypothesized that non-celiac gluten sensitivity might exist. Dr. Peter Gibson, a gastroenterologist at Monash University in Victoria, Australia, and his colleagues studied people with irritable bowel syndrome who did not have celiac disease but reacted badly to wheat. Many of the subjects still had symptoms on a gluten-free diet, and that prompted a second study of thirty-seven patients with both irritable bowel syndrome and non-celiac gluten sensitivity who were randomly assigned to a two-week diet, called FODMAPs, that is low in certain carbohydrates .

All patients on the special diet improved, but got significantly worse when fed gluten. Only 8 percent of the participants reacted specifically to gluten, prompting the researchers to conclude that FODMAPs, not gluten, accounted for most of the distress.

"FODMAPs" is an acronym for fermentable oligosaccharides, disaccharides, monosaccharides, and polyols, which are sugars that draw water into the intestinal tract. They may be poorly digested or absorbed, and so they become fodder for colonic bacteria that produce gas and can cause abdominal distress. They are:

- **Fructose:** A sugar prominent in apples, pears, watermelon, mangoes, grapes, blueberries, tomatoes and tomato concentrate, all dried fruits, vegetables (like sugar-snap peas, sweet peppers, and pickles), honey, agave, and jams, dressings, and drinks made with high-fructose corn syrup.
- **Lactose:** The sugar in milk from cows, goats, and sheep, which is also present in ice cream, soft cheeses, sour cream, and custard.
- **Fructans:** Soluble fiber found in bananas, garlic, onions, leeks, artichokes, asparagus, beets, wheat, and rye.
- **Galactans:** Complex sugars prominent in dried peas and beans, soybeans, soy milk, broccoli, cabbage, and brussels sprouts.
- **Polyols:** The sugar alcohols (sweeteners) isomalt, mannitol, sorbitol, and xylitol present in stone fruits like avocado, cherries, peaches, plums, and apricots.

People with irritable bowel syndrome often find that their symptoms lessen or disappear when avoiding foods rich in FODMAPs; however, it can take six to eight weeks on a low-FODMAP diet to see a significant improvement. The theory behind the low-FODMAP diet is that people with irritable bowel syndrome do not make enough of the enzymes that properly digest those five sugars. When the foods are eliminated, the symptoms go away.

Experts advise patients to eliminate all foods rich in FODMAPs at the start. (You can find a FODMAPs chart in the back of this book.) Once symptoms resolve, return individual foods to the diet, one by one, to identify those to which you react.

It has been my experience that clients with IBS do not stick with a traditional diet plan for long. Perhaps it is because the FODMAPs on it suddenly cause gas and bloating, and people assume the diet itself caused it, so they give up. The neat thing about the FODMAP chart is that you can use it to modify your diet plan, whatever nutritional plan you may be on, to eliminate the things you should not have and add the things that do not irritate you.

Adjusting to the menu may take awhile. Be patient with yourself. You will discover that some foods with bother you much more than others. When I saw the FODMAP chart for the first time, my first thought was, "I could have written it!" Most people with IBS do know most of the foods that bother them.

Here are some great resources for people with IBS using the FODMAP chart:

- http://www.ibsgroup.org/brochures/fodmap-intolerances.pdf
- https://beamingwithhealth.au.com/sites/default/files/download/LOWFODMAP.pdf
- http://www.katescarlata.com/

To Go Against the Grain or Not—That Is the Question

Gluten is the gluey protein found in grains like wheat, rye, barley, and malt. The signs of gluten sensitivity often mimic those of celiac disease, as well as irritable bowel syndrome. However, the man that helped make gluten-free diets popular, Dr. Peter Gibson, of FODMAP fame, admitted in May 2014 that he may have gotten it wrong. It may not have been the gluten causing that gastric distress after all! Further research showed it was the sugars in the bread that were hard to digest, not the gluten, caused the problem. (Google it for yourself!) Why has this news been buried in the press? Because the gluten-free fad has quickly become a billion-dollar industry!

One question I get asked frequently is whether or not someone should go gluten-free. Just like you probably have, I have read *Wheat Belly* by Dr. William Davis, and *Grain Brain* by Dr. David Perlmutter, and every other diet book out there. As someone who *cannot* eat wheat, I can't for the life of me figure out why people who *can* would deprive themselves of that delicious food. Many people go gluten-free to increase their energy level, but just eating more vegetables and fruits and *limiting* starches gives you tons of energy without having to totally do without gluten. We have a gluten-free Belly Buster Diet, but frankly, our clients get just as much of an increase in energy levels on the other menus.

As far as the irritation in the gut, ask your doctor to test you and prove that you have the irritation in your gut first before going to the extreme of this fad diet. And it *is* an extreme, it *is* a fad, and most people don't know how to properly do it because they don't have enough knowledge about nutrition to safely do it on their own. Most of my gluten-free clients do not stick to it as well as other clients on our other types of menus.

Here are four reasons to go gluten-free and four reasons not to. Make up your own mind what is best for you.

Reasons for Going Gluten-Free

1) **Managing celiac disease:** With this autoimmune disease, even trace amounts of gluten cause the immune system to attack the small intestine and cause significant damage. Unmanaged and under repeated attack, the intestines lose ability to absorb nutrients, which puts you at risk for developing other autoimmune disorders and problems.

2) **Controlling dermatitis herpetiformis (DH):** DH is a form of celiac disease that attacks the skin rather than the small intestine. Chronic itchy rashes that are symmetrical on each side of the body show up after eating gluten. If you have DH, you are at higher risk of intestinal cancer if you continue to eat gluten.

3) **Reducing the symptoms of gluten sensitivity:** These symptoms range from a wheat allergy to irritable bowel syndrome to just gas and bloating. When you do an elimination diet and the symptoms go away, you may feel so much better that you know it is the right thing to do. However, the FODMAP diet, where only some grains are omitted, may be a better choice.

4) **Supporting a family member who *has* to go gluten-free:** This makes it easier to cook and shop for the household.

Reasons for *Not* Going Gluten-Free

1) **Losing weight:** Gluten-free is probably the hardest diet to lose weight on because it is not easy to stick to, it is expensive, and most gluten-free products are high in carbs. Also, many gluten-free products are processed foods versus their counterparts that are natural whole foods. Gluten-free is tricky to do without missing important nutrients in your diet if you are not trained.

2) **Eating healthier:** It isn't healthier unless you are specifically going gluten-free to manage a particular medical condition. How are you replacing the fiber you are

losing? Are you getting enough? How about the carbohydrate intake? Do you know how much you need for your weight and activity level, and how much is safe to lose for your medical condition? Is a dietitian, nutritionist, or weight loss professional supervising you? Know what you are doing before you decide.

3) **Diagnosing your symptoms:** Don't do gluten-free to find out on your own. See a doctor for an accurate diagnosis while you are still eating a normal diet. The blood test used to diagnose celiac disease and DH depends on finding antibodies for gluten in your blood but it won't if you have avoided gluten.

4) **Because your best friend went gluten-free.** Chances are she/he won't last on it long, and when the next shiny object comes along, she/he will be jumping on that fad, too. Go with your gut (no pun intended). If you want to go gluten-free, make sure you can afford this expensive diet, can live totally without wheat and other foods you have to give up rather than simply cut back on them, can live with the inconvenience and can learn enough about nutrition that you truly feel comfortable doing it.

Just understand that going gluten-free is not necessary for most people and that research does not support the many theories behind it. In other words, it is just today's fad diet. There are no short cuts to a balanced, healthy lifestyle.

TIP: Read *Diet Cults* by Matt Fitzgerald for his perspective.

NOTES:_____

_____

_____

_____

_____

_____

_____

9 HANDLING HOLIDAYS

Fall may seem like a tough time to lose weight, but I've always found it easier than other times of year. Despite Halloween and Thanksgiving, you can lose a few pounds before the December holidays with these five fall tips.

1) **Concentrate on what you should and can have, not what you should not or cannot have.** Fall presents a delightful new cornucopia of foods that are great for dieting. Pumpkin can be used in recipes as a substitution for oil and is very low in carbs. Pumpkin soup with a little carrot shaved in it is much lower in carbs than acorn squash, and you can make it yourself with a low-fat chicken broth. You can make a baked apple instead of apple pie. Chop a whole unpeeled orange in the food processor with a bag of fresh cranberries and a few nuts for a delicious cranberry relish with one-third of the carbs of canned jellied cranberry sauce.

2) **Don't watch reality weight loss shows while you are trying to lose weight.** Those shows can set you up for failure because not many of us can work out five or six hours a day with our own private dietitian and personal

trainer. Our weight loss regime is not "made for TV"; instead, it's done one week at a time on a much smaller scale. Slow and easy is much better for a permanent fix.

3) **Fall is the perfect time to change up your exercise routine.** Most of us are more inclined to exercise outdoors when it is cooler. Something as simple as walking briskly, swimming, or biking for just twenty minutes three times per week will pick up your metabolism enough to lose an extra pound each week.

4) **Stay hydrated.** It is easy to drink water when it's hot; but when it's chilly outside, we don't always drink as much. To lose weight, you need to flush the melted fat. If you are used to drinking ice-cold water, perhaps switch to tepid water or flavored water that is not very cold. Switch it up. On cool fall nights, try a spiced tea and add green tea to it.

5) **Traditional holiday foods don't have to be fattening ones.** Think thin! Turkey, green beans, and pumpkin are *not* fattening foods—it is what *you* do to it that is! Look online to find recipes to adapt to your diet. There are great ones out there if you are serious about your health and making your body the best it can be. Some of my favorites are:

- http://lowcarb.betterrecipes.com
- http://www.hungry-girl.com/recipes
- www.bellybusterbabe.blogspot.com (my blog)

Here is my favorite fall dessert. It is great for Halloween or Thanksgiving or Christmas. It is made with Walden Farms products (which you can purchase through our clinics or at some grocers), and it doesn't taste like a diet recipe. Sonya Clemons-Baird adapted this pumpkin pie recipe from her family recipe for our clients.

Sonya's Turtle Pumpkin Pie
Crust:
Crush Melba toast and mix with 3 tablespoon Sugar-free Walden Farms Caramel Dip; press in bottom of 8x8 glass pan sprayed with cooking spray.
Topping:
Mix 3 tablespoons Walden Farms Marshmallow Dip with a

small container of Cool Whip. The whole thing will taste like marshmallows!

Pie:

3/4 c. Egg Beaters (or 3 eggs)
1 cup fat-free milk or plain soy milk
1/2 can pumpkin
2 packets of Before and After vanilla crème pudding mix *or* 2
  scoops of protein powder
1 teaspoon of pumpkin pie spice
16 pecan halves
Walden Farms Marshmallow Dip
Walden Farms Chocolate Syrup

In a blender, combine Egg Beaters, milk, pumpkin, pudding mix, and pumpkin pie spice. It will be thick. Pour over crust and bake at 350 degrees for 30 minutes. Cool in the refrigerator until completely chilled, then serve with two pecan halves crumbled over each serving with a tablespoon of marshmallow dip and chocolate syrup drizzled over it.

Another fall favorite is anything with apples. Nothing is more American than apple pie; but when you are dieting, even a plain medium apple can have a lot of carbs. On most low-carb diets, apples are either left out or you may have half an apple per day. However, I know a little secret I am going to share: mix cooked apples half and half with chayote, a South American squash, that you can get at any farmer's market. When you bake chayote with cinnamon and nutmeg, it tastes just like apples and it saves a lot of carbs. Chayote is a root vegetable that only has 11 grams of carbohydrates, while a medium apple has 21 grams of carbohydrates. When they're cooked, you cannot tell the difference—and they cost less, too!

I love Braeburn (sweet) and Granny Smith (tart) for baking, but with more than 25 varieties of apples to choose from, which you prefer will depend upon your palate. Your apples should be firm, crisp, vibrant in color, and not soft when you apply fingernail-pressure to the skin. If you are maintaining your weight, you can use the recipe listed here with apples and may even venture out and add white cheddar cheese over it if you like cheese with your apple pie or top it with just a little low-fat ice milk or frozen yogurt. For those of you who are in the battle of the bulge, I think you will love this chayote version of apple pie for the holidays with fresh (not canned) cranberries, which are also very low in carbs. The sugar-free jelly over it is optional, but it does add a wonderful sweetness and beautiful glaze, and it does not add very many calories or carbs. Enjoy!

Apple Cranberry Crisp
4 packets of protein oatmeal
¼ cup I Can't Believe It's Not Butter!
½ cup plain soy milk
4 medium apples or 5 chayotes (or a mixture of the two), peeled, cored, and sliced thick
½ teaspoon ground cinnamon
1 packet of sweetener
½ bag (about 2 cups) cranberries
1/3 jar (about 6 tablespoons) sugar-free apricot preserves

Preheat oven to 350 degrees. Spray a 9x13 dish, then melt the diet butter in it. Pour the oatmeal over the butter, and then pour just enough of the soy milk over it to cover the oats. Slice the apples on top, and then lightly dust with cinnamon and sweetener. Toss the fresh cranberries on top of the apples. Put dollops of the preserves over the top of the cranberries and bake for 45 to 55 minutes.

Variation for the holidays: Individual apples cored and baked and stuffed with the mixture make a great side dish or dessert for the holidays. These look so pretty on a plate with holly or greenery. Topped with frozen vanilla yogurt or whipped cream, it is sure to be a hit.

Tips for Handling the Holidays
If you are watching your weight *or* on a diet (yes, there is a difference), the holidays can be the time many give up or get discouraged. These belly bustin' holiday tips can help you get through the holidays and make you more conscious of what you are doing. First of all, don't see the holidays as a six-week long celebration; instead, see it as two or three special days. Give yourself permission to enjoy the individual holidays, but treat the in-between time like any other days of the year.

Be prepared: Some foods, especially those high in starch, act almost like a natural sedative. Knowing what sets you off will help you avoid a holiday binge. If you know that fudge or chocolate chip cookies are something you keep eating and eating as long as it is around, do not keep them in the house. I repeat: *Do not keep them in the house!* Take note of your emotional state, and do not eat when upset, depressed, or angry. Perhaps put that on an index card somewhere to remind you not to eat until your emotions in check. So instead of diving into food after a squabble with a relative, drink a glass of water or go for a brisk walk. Have a strategy ahead of time.

One meal at a time: If you lose control one day and eat ten sugar cookies, just remember that if you slip, it's not the end; it's just an occurrence. Tell yourself, "Tomorrow is another day, I'll get right back on my plan." The next day, follow your current weight loss plan and increase your protein intake. Don't decide your diet is a complete failure and throw in the towel before January 1. You have a goal! Keep the promise to yourself. Focus on what you want, not what you don't want.

TIP: Some dieters feel that if they blow their diet early in the day, they have already cheated so they give themselves permission to cheat the rest of the day. To keep yourself from doing that, get a calendar and a packet of gold and red stars and give yourself a gold star for every day you are good all day long and a red star for the days you struggled but got right back on track after a cheat. You will soon be tackling your diet one meal at the time instead of letting it ruin your whole day if you can't stick to it.

Parties—plan ahead: Before the office parties and family get-togethers, set aside a time to mentally focus on how you'd like to handle the occasion. For a couple of days before the event, set aside five minutes a day to visualize the event: who you'll be with, how you'll act, what you'll eat, and what you'll talk about. If you can see yourself acting the way you wish to behave, you're more likely to behave that way at the event itself.

When you are going to a party, plan ahead of time what you are going to do about drinking. If you drink a full glass of water in between each glass of alcohol, that will help flush out some of the alcohol; plus, it will help fill you up. Just make sure water will be available or take it with you. Also, plan your strategy for eating at the party.

TIP: Fill up on protein first with things like cheese, shrimp cocktail, crab dip, meat roll-ups, or little smokies before eating any sweets or drinking alcohol. Protein will help stabilize your blood sugar and will help carbs and fruit sugars break down more slowly. You will not drink as much or consume as many carbohydrates and blow your diet.

Practice "no": When you are dieting, saying "no" shows that you are in control. If you have friends who are also trying to lose weight, and they can't resist, they will want a partner in crime. Don't let other peoples' need to indulge cause you to indulge also. Instead of just saying "no" whenever someone asks why you're not trying this or that, just say, "I am stuffed! I ate a huge meal earlier." Most people won't take "no" for an answer, but this is a "no" most people understand, and they'll drop it.

You—The Party Giver
Don't keep holiday treats around after the party, or they will end up being your snack food. Make sure you send all your guests out the door with a food gift. You can also make things that you can freeze for the next party.

Food tends to be the focal point of most celebrations, but it doesn't have to be. Add candles, flowers, or music to add to the holiday atmosphere. More important, remember that the holidays are not about turkey, ham, and desserts as much as being about bringing friends and family together.

Prepare foods at your parties for both dieters and non-dieters. You will find many holiday recipes on our clinics' blog, www.bellybusterbabe.blogspot.com.

Here is a recipe that I especially like for parties. It's quick and easy:

No-Bake Chocolate Truffles
2 tablespoons PB2
1 tablespoon water
Mix well according to package directions.
2 teaspoon cocoa powder
½ banana or 2 tablespoons pumpkin (go by what is on your diet)
½ cup oatmeal *or* 2 packets of oatmeal protein supplement

Mix all ingredients with the first two and add water a little at the time if more is needed. Roll into one-inch balls and place on waxed cookie sheet. You can roll them in coconut or nuts for guests who are not dieting.

You can also make these with pumpkin, oatmeal, PB2, pumpkin pie spice, and water and roll in crushed pepitas. If your protein supplement does not have dried apples in it, add applesauce or apples diced finely.

RECPES:_____

_____

_____

_____

_____

_____

_____

_____

_____

_____

_____

_____

_____

_____

_____

_____

_____

_____

NOTES:_____

_____

_____

_____

_____

_____

_____

_____

_____

_____

_____

_____

What are your biggest challenges during the holidays?_____

_____

_____

_____

_____

How can you overcome them while dieting?_____

_____

_____

_____

10 HANDLING PLATEAUS

Not many people can diet without reaching a plateau at some point. Unfortunately, that is the point at which most people give up. However, plateaus are only a sign to change up what you are doing, *not* a sign to quit! Once you understand the many reasons you stop losing weight *temporarily* and the ways you can jump-start weight loss, you won't have any reason to stop your journey. First and foremost, you have to be honest with yourself: Are you truly sticking to your nutritional plan with *no* exceptions? Make a list of the foods and other things you have had in your mouth over the past few days that were not on the plan. Add up the carbs and calories. Be sure to include over-the-counter products like Pepto-Bismol, Tums, NyQuil, and chocolate calcium chews, and also count chewing gum if it contains more than 1 gram of carbohydrates.

Here is an example of extra things someone might eat in a day and not count on their food plan: You are cleaning the table after breakfast, and Little Johnnie didn't eat all of his waffle or drink all of his chocolate milk, so you finish it for him; you have this thing about throwing food away. You make Little Johnnie's sandwich for school and he wants the crusts cut off of his peanut butter and jelly sandwich. You cut them off and eat them. "It's just the crust," you tell yourself. You get to work and the boss has M&M's on his desk. You eat just a handful, not many. At lunch, you order a salad with vinaigrette dressing and take off the croutons—you are so proud of yourself! You stick to your diet at dinner, except that you are eating out and the bread in the restaurant is *not* on your program. Since you are supposed to have bread at dinner, you eat it anyway. On the way home, you think you have done well on your diet, so you have two Jolly Ranchers as a reward as your husband asks, "How's the diet working for you, Hon?" Then, you tell your counselor at your next weigh-in that you have no idea why you are not losing weight.

Let's add up the extra calories in this day:

½ waffle	70 calories
¼ cup chocolate milk	60 calories
crust on sandwich	70 calories
M&M's	60 calories
vinaigrette dressing	90 calories
roll	100 calories more than diet bread
2 Jolly Ranchers	50 calories
	500 calories

"Do your diet plan the way it is written, not the way you have modified it for yourself" —Michael Vernon, VP, Belly Buster Diet, Inc.

Are you willing to do the exercise it will take to burn the extra 500 calories? It takes six hundred push-ups or sixty minutes of jumping jacks or jazzercise. Or how about snorkeling for an hour and 20 minutes? That sounds like so much more fun than forty-five minutes on the elliptical, doesn't it? Wouldn't it be simpler just to stick to your plan in the first place?

Self-Test For Determining the Cause of Slow Weight Loss
1) Do you drink enough water to flush the melted fat and toxins from your body? (When dieting, you should drink about 64 ounces for the first 200 pounds and about 8 ounces for every 25 pounds over 200.)
2) Have you recently changed medications?
3) Have you recently eaten anything salty or eaten out and

don't know the sodium content of what you ate?

4) Are you having hormone fluctuations at this time?

5) Are you constipated and straining when you go to the bathroom?

6) Are you using the correct amount and kind of protein required on your program?

7) Are you using the correct amount and kind of oil and fats for your program?

8) Are you using the correct amount of carbohydrates for your program (i.e., fruits, vegetables, and starches)?

9) Are you using the correct amount of bread and fiber for your particular plan?

10) Are you eating fresh fruits and vegetables and limiting canned varieties, like tuna or crushed pineapple, to occasional consumption?

11) Are you eating deli meats that are low sodium and that are not prepackaged?

12) Are you avoiding juice and eating whole fruits instead?

13) Are you eating your servings of fruit only before 3:00 p.m.?

14) Are you eating main meals four to five hours apart?

15) Are you going to bed at least three hours after eating?

16) Are you varying your foods?

17) Are you weighing and measuring your food?

18) Are you removing skin from poultry before you eat it?

19) Are you watching how often you eat meats and seafood with higher cholesterol? (In the Belly Buster Diet, these foods are called Group B meats.)

20) Are you eating the correct number of meals a day for your diet plan?

21) Are you leaving off the foods that are not allowed? Review them with your coach to be sure. What may be right for one plan may not biochemically be right for another.

22) Are you avoiding tasting while cooking?

23) Do you avoid using too many artificial sweeteners?

24) If your plan calls for soy milk or almond milk, do you use *unflavored*? (The flavored adds lots of sugar and calories!)

25) Do you limit the number of times you have nutritional bars? (You may want to give them up until you are off the

plateau. Most have a lot of carbs.)
26) Have you recently taken antibiotics? (You can avoid the weight gain and plateau with a round of antibiotics by taking probiotics with them.)
27) Have you limited the amount of tomatoes and tomato sauces you are eating?
28) Have you checked the carbs of the chewing gum and mints you use?
29) Have you cut back or preferably stopped drinking alcohol while dieting?
30) Have you checked the carb content of your salad dressings?

If you have answered all thirty of these questions and find more than four or five things you need to change, modify your behavior. If you find fewer than three or four things you can change, try one of the following plateau breakers. These are tried-and-true methods of breaking plateaus that have worked for thousands of clients in our clinics.

Plateau Breakers
Here are six plateau breakers you can do to break a period of no weight loss. Usually the first one works within just a few days. If you complete one and it doesn't break the plateau, don't repeat the same one. Pick a different one to try, and have confidence one of these will work.
1) **4-2-3-1.** Vary the number of protein supplements you are taking (hence 4-2-3-1) and vary your foods as much as possible. Repeat twice for a total of eight days. Sometimes you are on a plateau because you eat the same food at each meal every day. Shake it up a little bit! Your body needs a variety of nutrients. If your nutritional plan does not call for protein supplements, try incorporating them for plateaus. If you are on one that does, be sure to use their brand because they have chosen them for a reason.
2) **Increase your oil.** You can use oil in your salad dressing by mixing 1 tablespoon canola oil and 1 tablespoon apple cider vinegar and seasonings without salt. Both of these help you lose weight. Canola oil has much more CLA in it than olive oil does, and the apple cider will help emulsify

fat. Increase your dose of flaxseed capsules from three to six per day or EFA from two to three per day, if you take those. (Note: If you are on blood thinners, ask before you take flax or EFA, and don't increase them if you take Serrapeptase or Trim N Shape daily.) If you are constipated, take psyllium or sienna tea first, and then take EFA. The oil will help you stay regular, but oil is not taken for constipation per se.

3) **Take digestive enzymes.** You can get them from our clinic for just $15 per bottle or at any health food store. Take one per day with breakfast or lunch for two weeks to break a plateau. *Do not* take longer than two weeks or within two weeks of a blood test, as it will give false readings for elevated liver enzymes. This strategy is good for those with slow digestion, older clients, and women with three or more children. Older clients may want to take enzymes often.

4) **Go back to preconditioning if you are on the Belly Buster Diet.** *Only do this after discussing it with your consultant.* This is good if you have been off program, cheated, or been on vacation, but it is best not to do it more than every three months. Be sure to restart with your initial menu when you finish preconditioning (if on the Belly Buster Diet, it will be the Cream or O, B, G, or L series or you can do whatever series you were on). If you are on another diet, we strongly recommend that you do not do colon cleansers, but instead do something similar to our detox menu. Eat lots of fiber, fruits, and vegetables, and very little meat. That will naturally cleanse the colon, whereas colon cleanser systems or pills tend to strip the cilia, the hairs in the intestines, of their ability to pick up nutrients.

5) **Increase your exercise.** While you need to walk, doing it slowly doesn't help a whole lot. It may be time to actually sweat a little! Go to the treadmill or do a more fast-paced walk. If you're swimming, try increasing laps. If you're biking, try longer distances or a faster pace. Try a video dance or walk tape or DVD.

6) **Try the Plateau Breaker menu available in the clinic.** It has the lowest-carb foods on our menu, and five protein

supplements a day for five days. This is good if you have not been doing at least three protein supplements a day; two is the minimum, but you don't usually plateau with three. For any other nutritional plans, try carb cycling. Cycle from eating three to four days of low-carb to one to two days of no carbs and then a high-carb diet for one day. Some simple plans have one day of low carb and one day of high carb, but the basic idea is to alternate the carbohydrate content of your food intake to confuse the metabolism. Some people may find it hard to do all the time for a diet because once you taste that pasta or pizza, you may want it too often. However, it is great for breaking a plateau or for that last pesky 10 pounds. If you search for carb cycling online, make sure you are on a reputable site because several I checked listed high-carb vegetables to eat on the days you were to eat low-carb foods. If you are on the Belly Buster Diet, you can use the preconditioning menu as your high-carb cycle. Flip between that menu and your diet menu rather than guessing which foods you should use.

NOTES:_____

_____

_____

_____

_____

_____

_____

_____

_____

_____

_____

—

SECTION II:
THE EMOTIONAL PART
OF EATING

Introduction to Life Choices with Michael Vernon

This section of the book is written by my partner, Michael Vernon, a behavioral scientist who teaches Choose Your Life, Choose Your Destiny Classes (aka, Life Choices) at our Before ad After Weight Loss Clinics on the Treasure Coast of Florida. We feel so strongly about his material that we only guarantee our program if our clients attend his course on the emotional part of eating.

"Doing the same thing over and over and over again and expecting change, without a change in the process, is a sign of insanity."—Albert Einstein

Nancy Lee McCaskill & Michael Vernon

11 EMOTIONAL BOUNDARIES

Putting everyone else's needs and desires ahead of yours is quite common. It is a reflection of your love for your family and neighbors, isn't it? Is that good or bad? How can loving your family be bad? It is bad only if you have stopped loving yourself in the process. Does anyone take advantage of you and your time? If so, draw your line in the sand.

Is thinking of yourself first selfish? Now, that is a good question. It is a matter of perspective, to be sure. On one hand, giving of yourself and of your time can make you feel good; but on the other hand, if *you* are not healthy, how can you be there for others?

A good example is a commercial airplane ride. The flight attendants go over a few rules before you lift off. First, this is your seat belt and this is how you fasten it. Next, the closest exit may be behind you. Take a few moments to find the exit nearest you; and if the cabin fills with smoke, the arrows on the floor will direct you to the exit. Should the cabin lose air pressure, a mask will fall from the compartment above you: "Please put yours on first before helping the person next to you."

This is the time to put "you" higher on the totem pole. That way you can ensure that you are able to be there for others, and you can show others how to treat you by how you treat yourself.

Make sense?

You set boundaries all the time. Family almost always comes ahead of strangers; but what about your family and you personally? Do everyone's needs and desires come before yours, or do you set some boundaries there as well? Are some boundaries good when it comes to your health? In certain circumstances, are you willing to bend your boundaries for others in your life? Where do you draw the line?

Emergencies, for sure, may be a good reason. The busiest person I know has a sign above his desk that simply reads, "Poor planning on your part doesn't necessarily constitute an emergency on mine." He gives a little wiggle room for those he cares for. If you were bleeding or having a heart attack, he would drop everything and come to your assistance. That is what any good friend would do. Emergencies are about the only things that can get him off his focus. That is how he gets things done. He has had tremendous success in his life and still enjoys it as well as anyone without jumping at the whim of everyone else.

Are you a people-pleaser who finds it hard to increase your emotional boundaries? Some people find it easier than others. But doing so will help you maintain focus, avoid distractions, and help you have more time to find nonfood-related ways of rewarding yourself for your good behavior.

Nevertheless, life does get in the way sometimes, tempting us to abandon our emotional boundaries. The thought paradigm each of us is made of allows us to fall back on a subconscious level in ways that we are not even aware of most of the time and don't even feel. Life throws things at us daily, such as codependent relationships disguised as "obligations" that we have to deal with on some level or another. The following story is an example of that and has come in handy time and time again to demonstrate how easy it is to fall back into old patterns and lose focus on what our true goals are.

This fable by Rabbi Edwin Friedman, "The Bridge," is in Peter Scazzero's book _The Emotionally Healthy Church: A Strategy for Discipleship That Actually Changes Lives_. The chapter is called "Receiving the Gift of Limits". As you read this story, imagine yourself as the main character. Have a friend read this and discuss it with you. Take the time to reread it when a situation comes up for you when you don't need to "hold the rope". If you are a people-pleaser, make a copy of it and read it frequently! Think about how many times in your life you have held the rope for others and how you now react differently.

The Bridge

Rabbi Edwin Friedman tells the story of a man who had given much thought to what he wanted from life. After trying many things, succeeding at some and failing at others, he finally decided what he wanted.

One day the opportunity came for him to experience exactly the way of living that he had dreamed about. But the opportunity would be available only for a short time. It would not wait, and it would not come again.

Eager to take advantage of this open pathway, the man started on his journey. With each step, he moved faster and faster. Each time he thought about his goal, his heart beat quicker; and with each vision of what lay ahead, he found renewed vigor.

As he hurried along, he came to a bridge that crossed through the middle of a town. The bridge spanned high above a dangerous river.

After starting across the bridge, he noticed someone coming from the opposite direction. The stranger seemed to be coming toward him to greet him. As the stranger grew closer, the man could discern that they didn't know each other, but yet they looked amazingly similar. They were even dressed alike. The only difference was that the stranger had a rope wrapped many times around his waist. If stretched out, the rope would reach a length of perhaps thirty feet.

The stranger began to unwrap the rope as he walked. Just as the two men were about to meet, the stranger politely said, "Pardon me, would you be so kind as to hold the end of the rope for me?"

The man agreed without a thought, reached out, and took it.

"Thank you," said the stranger. He then added, "Two hands now, and remember, hold tight." At that point, the stranger jumped off the bridge.

The man on the bridge abruptly felt a strong pull from the now-extended rope. He automatically held tight and was almost dragged over the side of the bridge.

"What are you trying to do?" he shouted to the stranger below.

"Just hold tight," said the stranger.

This is ridiculous, the man thought. He began trying to haul the other man in. Yet it was just beyond his strength to bring the other back to safety.

Again he yelled over the edge, "Why did you do this?"

"Remember," said the other, "if you let go, I will be lost."

"But I cannot pull you up," the man cried.

"I am your responsibility," said the other.

"I did not ask for it," the man said.

"If you let go, I am lost," repeated the stranger.
The man began to look around for help. No one was within sight.
He began to think about his predicament. Here he was eagerly pursuing a unique opportunity, and now he was being sidetracked for who knows how long. Maybe I can tie the rope somewhere, he thought. He examined the bridge carefully, but there was no way to get rid of his newfound burden. So he again yelled over the edge, "What do you want?"
"Just your help," came the answer.
"How can I help? I cannot pull you in, and there is no place to tie the rope while I find someone else who could help you."
"Just keep hanging on," replied the dangling man. "That will be enough."
Fearing that his arms could not hold out much longer, he tied the rope around his waist.
"Why did you do this?" he asked again. "Don't you see who you have done? What possible purpose could you have in mind?"
"Just remember," said the other, "my life is in your hands."
Now the man was perplexed. He reasoned within himself: If I let go, all my life I will know that I let this other man die. If I stay, I risk losing my momentum toward my own long-sought-after salvation. Either way this will haunt me forever.
As time went by, still no one came. The man became keenly aware that it was almost too late to resume his journey. If he didn't leave immediately, he wouldn't arrive in time.
Finally, he devised a plan. "Listen," he explained to the man hanging below, "I think I know how to save you." He mapped out the idea. The stranger could climb back up by wrapping the rope around him. Loop by loop, the rope would become shorter.
But the dangling man had no interest in the idea.
"I don't think I can hang on much longer," warned the man on the bridge.
"You must try," appealed the stranger. "If you fail, I die."
Suddenly a new idea struck the man on the bridge. It was different and even alien to his normal way of thinking. "I want you to listen carefully," he said, "because I mean what I am about to say."
The dangling man indicated that he was listening.
"I will not accept the position of choice for your life, only for my own; I hereby give back the position of choice for your own life to you."
"What do you mean?" the other asked, afraid.
"I mean, simply, it's up to you. You decide which way this ends. I will become the counterweight. You do the pulling and bring yourself up. I will even tug some from here."

He unwound the rope from around his waist and braced himself to be a counterweight. He was ready to help as soon as the dangling man began to act.

"You cannot mean what you say," the other shrieked. "You would not be so selfish. I am your responsibility. What could be so important that you would let someone die? Do not do this to me."

After a long pause, the man on the bridge uttered slowly, "I accept your choice." In voicing those words, he freed his hands and continued his journey over the bridge.

Could you have done that? Could you let go? How many codependent relationships do you have? How many times have you not let go and fallen back instead of moving forward?

You are not here to fix all of the world's problems. You can't do it all, and you can't allow other people's expectations make you feel guilty. You have take care of yourself first and foremost, without making yourself fell guilty either. Remember the airplane oxygen mask? Remember the "you only get one car so you have to take care of it" story?

First, start with small changes. Some very simple changes in the way you think can have a big impact on your diet. For instance, the word *diet* has two good meanings. If your doctor would ask you about your diet, he or she is asking about your overall food intake. We, on the other hand, think of a *diet* as a temporary change in eating habits to lose excess weight. Somewhere in the back of your mind you are probably still thinking you will go back to the way you used to eat before the diet. But you will never be able to completely go back to the way you used to eat because that's what got you to where you didn't want to be in the first place. Just like Einstein said, something has to change or you will do things over and over with the same results.

Subconsciously, the word *diet* can have a negative connotation. After all, the word *diet* has the word *die* at the beginning of it. Try this: Find a different word, other than *diet*, to describe your food intake. How do these sound: new meal plan, menu planner, or nutritional program? Just find one that is best for you. "This is my new nutritional program for the rest of my long, healthy, and happy life." Sound better? It reaffirms why you are eating healthier every time you say it.

Next, develop a clear vision of your motivation. Whatever it is, it has to be bigger than any excuse you can come up with for not doing it. Your *why* has to be bigger than your *but*. Humans can rationalize nearly *anything* they want to justify satisfying a perceived immediate need. More will be discussed on that in chapter thirteen, "Food Addiction".

"Getting anything you want in life is as simple as the A, B, C's...if you have a great attitude, a strong belief that you can do it and an unshakable commitment to your goal, you can do almost anything, even fly in space and land on the Moon." —June Scobee, wife of *Challenger* commander Richard Scobee

Finally, understand which time bandits steal your personal time. Don't try and solve everyone's problems, but be there for the emergencies. That is what friends do. Be sure to respect yourself and find time for you, first and foremost. Your emotions are your emotions, and it is OK to have them. You have a right to have them, but it is your responsibility to control how you respond to other people's emotions. It's not good for your well-being to get enmeshed in others' emotions and feelings. You can feel, however, that you want to be responsible for everything you do feel and for how you react, regardless of what other people think, say, or do. Bottom line, no one can make you happy, mad, glad, or sad but you. Emotional eating does not happen because someone *made* you feel a certain way. No one does that to you but *you*!

It is all right to be empathetic, even a bit sympathetic, but don't let others steer you off your plan to achieve your goals and aspirations. Recognize what triggers your emotions and develop coping mechanisms to deal with these triggers in order to make your weight loss permanent. If you happen to have unshakable self-esteem, then you may already know how to do what you need to do. If you don't, the following seven chapters/classes will help you have impeccable character with sterling integrity with a fit body and healthy lifestyle.

How did you feel about The Bridge story?

_____

_____

_____

12 CONTROL ISSUES

If nobody is holding you down and feeding you, then you are in control of what goes inside—or are you? Our subconscious controls us on a level we don't even know exists; but who put those thoughts there? Our parents? ("You can't leave the table until that plate is clean.") Our grandparents? ("I always like a little something sweet after dinner.") Our peers? ("Come on, I made it just for you!") What kind of self-talk do *you* use when you pass by a mirror? ("UGH! You are so fat!") Our subconscious mind is dictating these things to us every time we sit down at the table, confirming what we subconsciously believe.

We are also unintentionally trained from a very early age to use food to change our moods, and we revert to those comfort foods when conscious control eludes us. This results in emotional eating. When a baby cries, what happens? They either get picked up and cuddled, they get their diaper changed, or they get fed—all good things. Advance a bit further to ages 2 and 3. The child comes home upset, and we sit them down and give them a cookie; if it is a really bad situation, we give him a whole batch of cookies. Later on this emotional eating transforms into the freshman fifteen, the fifteen or so pounds some freshman college students gain because they are eating on their terms without the supervision of someone to tell them no.

Now, as adults we surely have control over what we make for our meals. Habitual eating comes from what our parents (or whoever raised us) taught us. The types of foods people like and how they prepare them are often passed down from generation to generation. So, is it our mother's fault? Well, that is somewhat true; but we are intelligent beings, and schools and nutritionists have been telling us about health problems associated with certain foods for years.

Regardless of age, the amount of food we eat is our choice, and there are a multitude of challenges to eating properly at different ages. During our growth years, it is hard to fill us up; and then, when we get to middle age, those patterns are hard to change, especially if no one points them out. In older age, we might even forget to eat sometimes.

Overeating is also easy to do because of today's world of fast-paced convenience and oversized portions. You grab a quick bite on the way to school or work. You eat at your desk because the overachievers are doing it, and you have to keep up. Then, after work you have an avalanche of activities. It doesn't help that you see hundreds of food commercials on TV, making it very hard to escape temptation.

Restaurants certainly don't help matters. Remember, they are in the food business to sell food. They want to make sure you are well satisfied and happy you came, so you come back time and time again. They want you to get your money's worth, so they will serve you two or three times a normal portion size without batting an eye. What would you think if you paid for a steak dinner and the plate came out with a 3-ounce portion for a lady or a 4- or 5-ounce portion for a man? Would you look at the server and ask, "Where's the beef?" Make it chicken, and you'll probably get two huge breasts on a bed of rice or pasta, which is enough for three meals at the proper portion sizes. Many restaurants even add endless bread or endless salad bars to go along with their huge portions.

TIP: When eating out, ask for a take-home box when your meal comes and divide your meal in half. You'll have a great lunch the next day. People will marvel at your discipline, and you will be making great progress towards you goal.

Is it any wonder why 67 percent of Americans are considered to be 10 to 20 pounds or more overweight and nearly 30 percent of adults are considered obese, or more than 30 pounds or more overweight?

No matter what your age, no matter what your situation, the one thing *you* can control is what and how much goes inside you. At times, you must be assertive to get food prepared the way you want it. Do not feel guilty because you have expressed your desires. Would you consider asking for the butter to be left off or the meat not to be fried to be assertive or controlling? Is there a difference? You can send a meal back in a way that is tasteful without being rude; but would you? Do you believe that you control how you respond to other people—friends, family, waitstaff—regardless of what they might say? If not, why not?

Awareness of your choices is half the battle. Once you become aware of your behavior and the ability to correct it, you should be able to find a course of direction that removes outside influences from dictating your choice. Understand that it is your choice, not because of anything else except your right to a choice.

"Your life is in your hands. No matter where you are now, no matter what has happened in your life, you can begin to consciously choose your thoughts, and you can change your life. There is no such thing as a hopeless situation. Every single circumstance of your life can change!" —Rhonda Byrne, author of *The Secret*

Other people can respond any way they want to because it is also their right to do so. You cannot control that, though you may want to. Want to know if you are controlling of others? That's easy—ask them; they know. There is a difference between assertive and controlling. Controlling people tend not to shy from confrontation and can be a bit pushy or manipulative. Assertive people generally avoid conscious manipulation and can be sensitive to others, but not to the point of being abused themselves or forsaking their needs and desires.

Is it OK to be a bit more passive? Sure, it is situationally dependent. A lot more passive? Nope, people won't stop loving if you are being a wimp most of the time, but standing up for yourself and showing others how to treat you by how you treat yourself can go a long way to improving your self-esteem. Once you begin voicing your needs and desires, nothing will seem out of the question or impossible.

Surrounding yourself with only good relationships is a great idea to help you take control of your choices. Positive, uplifting people tend to attract positive, uplifting people. Relationships with mutual respect are founded on the understanding that there can be more than one opinion at a time and that it is OK to agree to disagree. If you have naysayers among your group, focusing on mutual respect helps you understand that you cannot be all things to all people, and it is unreasonable to expect that of yourself. When you show respect for yourself it is much easier to gain respect from others.

How can you get past the conflicting motivations of people in your life and maintain the balance you need? Recognize each person's behavior—including your own—so you can position yourself appropriately and not give into energy-draining events and conflicts. For example: your spouse, mother, or father come at you with a criticism of a decision you made, "What were you thinking? How could you have done such a thing? You had no right to …" Get the point? Instead of feeling guilty of your decision, you let them know it was just that, *your* decision and, "Unless you were there in my shoes, it is a bit unfair of you to say that, don't you agree?" or "I made the best decision that I could with the information I had at the time."

It is up to each person how they deal with their interpersonal relationships. Intention is important to determining if they are being controlling or assertive. Have you ever slammed a door to make a point? Have you ever broken anything and then felt horrible about it because you caused the accident? Some people swear and throw things, and sometimes even hit things and people that get in their way. Ever fake a stomachache or headache to get out of something? Remember Fred Sanford from *Sanford and Son*? When his son Lamont did something Fred didn't like or if Fred wasn't included in Lamont's decision-making process, he grabbed his chest, faking a heart attack and claiming he was coming to "meet his Elizabeth in heaven," because it was the "big one". He was bit overdramatic just because he felt excluded and wanted to make a point. Have you ever controlled a situation by faking an illness or calling in sick?

In *The Celestine Prophecy*, James Redfield describes an unconscious competition for energy by humans as the source for conflict in the world. To get past it, he says we need to be filled with a sense of love. Then there will be no need to steal energy from others.

So, ask yourself a simple question: Do you love yourself? Remember the oxygen mask on the airplane: "Put yours on first before the person next to you." You show others how to treat you by how you treat yourself.

You cannot control everything in your life and you cannot control how others behave or what they say. Let go of that and let fate or karma deal with those things. Remember that other people have their own issues, control issues, anger issues, and programming issues, just like you. Control what goes on inside *you* and if you have a hard time of that, reprogram your self-talk by doing affirmations (see chapter eighteen "How to Do Affirmations"). Strive to make better choices, and you will do OK. Keep getting back up on the horse when you fall off. Even the best riders get knocked off sometimes. Your personal integrity is what is most important: Do what you say you are going to do when you say you are going to do it. Build on that and you will be unstoppable.

Who controls you? Who do you control?

_____

_____

_____

How does it affect what you eat---or does it?

_____

_____

_____

_____

_____

_____

NOTES:_____

13 FOOD ADDICTION

Are you addicted to food, or do you just love it? Do you eat to live or live to eat? Is food's importance to your life out of proportion? After all, we all have to eat, so shouldn't we have a healthy relationship with food?

Is there a food can you not live without? If you answer that you have a few that you cannot live without, you may be a full-blown food addict. Do you want to eat it because it makes you feel good? If some behavior doesn't make you feel good, it is unlikely you will do it over and over again, agreed? Think about the most common addictions like drugs, alcohol, sex, and gambling. All of them give us a little dose of *feel good* (dopamine) inside. If a little is good, more must be better; but too much can be a bad thing. Moderation becomes the key; and if the behavior starts to become an excuse, you just might be heading for a problem. It is best to deal with it sooner rather than later. Your friends and family will know if you have a problem; ask them. Or, in the case of food addiction, your belt buckle may tell you.

Moderation and portion control are the keys to maintaining your weight. Calories in and calories out, you consume too many calories and you will gain weight. Conversely, if you use or burn more calories than you take in, you will lose weight. However, if you are a food addict, who is counting? You become a master at justifying the calories and justifying the lack of exercise. We eat to provide nutrition for our minds and bodies; but why else might we eat? Sometimes we will eat as an emotional response. As we discussed earlier, it comforts us. Perhaps we eat out of boredom when there is nothing to do. Do you ever eat to get rid of feelings of loneliness or anxiety? Do you ever catch yourself eating seconds or thirds because the normal helping didn't fill you up? Do you ever feel a sense of being out of control because it was just so good you felt you couldn't get enough? Any and all of these can be a sign of trouble.

Eating disorders manifest as all kinds of behaviors and emotions. Our attempts to control them go from one extreme to the other. Fear of getting too big can lead to anorexia and bulimia, depending on diet pills, or one fad diet after another. Some will try to control weight by unnatural eating and purging, some with various pharmaceuticals, and some will go on a merry-go-round, never finding a comfortable relationship with food.

Not sure how healthy your relationship with food is? Count how many of the following excuses you have used to justify a bad food choice. It is important to remember that humans are pleasure-seekers; given a choice between a pleasurable activity and a tough one, we will go to the warm and comfy side most of the time.

I am eating unhealthy foods today because:

___I am on vacation.

___No one taught me how to make healthy foods.

___I was taught to clean my plate and it would be rude not to; it would insult the chef.

___It is the weekend. I always eat more and take a break on the weekend.

___Hey, it wouldn't be Thanksgiving without all the fixins.

___We always celebrate birthdays by eating out or making that person's favorite food.

___Every Sunday we meet at Granny's house and bring a dish. She cooks the main courses, and the rest of us bring the side dishes. We have done that for years and years.

___This stuff is on my diet, maybe not this much, but at least it is fat-free.

___I missed lunch today, so I am eating more now.

___I am eating more now, but I'll make it up by working out later.

___I am eating more because I worked hard today.

___I am eating off program (Campbell's soup) because I am sick.

See how easy it is? Any excuse can be good enough to let you off the hook for a little when you are looking for a reason. Is it ok to cheat on your diet? No, but we are human and not perfect. Just remember that the restrictive part of a diet is short term, a temporary solution to a permanent problem. You can do without anything for six weeks, right?

TIP: Get a calendar for your refrigerator and a pack of gold stars. Every day that you are absolutely true to your diet and keep your promise to yourself, give yourself a gold star. As simple as it is, this technique is a great low-cost technique to motivate yourself. If you absolutely have to have a cheat day, pick one day each month to eat anything you want. It can be a holiday, your birthday, an event, or the same day of the month each month. But eat reasonably and resist going overboard, and you will feel better about yourself. Your self-esteem is going to grow, and soon nothing will be able to stop you.

Don't beat yourself up if you flub up occasionally, but commit to trying harder and improving yourself until you adopt the new habits to maintain the new you. Keep the promises you make yourself no matter what—no matter how hard it may seem, no matter what life may throw your way—and it will become easier and easier.

Let's tackle those excuses one at a time.

"I am on vacation." Do you have to sample all of the local cuisine to have a full experience of the locale? Of course not. You can even lose weight on a cruise if you stick to your guns about what and how much you eat. Every cruise ship has a buffet with grilled or baked chicken and plenty of salads and vegetables. Most ships have light fare that actually tastes better than the regular courses. The main dining room and all the tempting desserts aren't a necessity. You can bank ahead of the event knowing you might indulge by working out or walking a few extra miles. You have a choice. Make the better choice every time, even when it is not a cruise, and you will do OK.

"No one taught me how to make healthy foods." Well, it is time to learn. Ignorance is bliss, but knowing better and not doing something about it isn't. There are plenty of websites and books available about how to make the foods that you love healthier for you. Experiment a little. healthy recipes on the Food Network It is fun, and you just might learn something. **TIP:** The blog for Belly Buster Diet is at https://bellybusterbabe.blogspot.com/, and we also love the (http://www.foodnetwork.com/healthy.html).

"I was taught to clean my plate and it would be rude not to; it would insult the chef." Times have changed since this mantra was popular. It was no doubt started by those who survived the Great Depression and World War II. Food was scarce then, and having a full plate was a luxury. There were no supermarkets or refrigerators. Today many homes have more than one fridge and a separate freezer. The supermarket is open 365 days a year with plenty of meats, fresh vegetables, and fruits. Canning has almost become a lost art. As for insulting the chef, it is OK to leave food on your plate if you were overserved. It is your choice what goes inside of you. Be strong, and others will honor you for your discipline.

"Hey, it wouldn't be Thanksgiving without all the fixins." Yes it would. Would it be so bad if you skipped just one all-day feast on Thanksgiving to eat proper portions? Four or five ounces of turkey breast, string beans, squash casserole, fresh cranberries, pumpkin pie—no problem. It is a problem if it becomes two or three helpings of pumpkin pie or a huge plateful of food drenched in gravy with three or four dinner rolls. Can you have one small bite to taste? Sure, if you can keep it to that without the mountain of guilt that might accompany it. Remember, balance is what you are trying achieve, and if you can put in a little extra exercise before, during, and after after Thanksgiving, you can *lightly* sample about anything you want on the special fourth Thursday of November. But beware: The average person puts on 10 pounds between Thanksgiving and New Year's because of all the food temptations during that holiday period. Skipping one year to reach your goal is not much to sacrifice. Keep your eyes on the prize and put the fork and spoon down just this once.

"We always celebrate birthdays by going out to eat or making that person's favorite food." Celebrating with food is a centuries-old tradition and one of the toughest food habits to break. However, you can eat healthy foods on birthdays and holidays if your goal is important enough to you! You will have another birthday next year, and you will be slimmer, but *not* if you keep using everyone's birthday and gathering as an excuse to veer off-course and eat whatever fattening thing appears at the next shindig. Keep it to a bite or two and save normal proper portion sizes for when you have reached your maintenance weight. There is always next year!

"Every Sunday we meet at Granny's house and bring a dish. She cooks the main courses, and the rest of us bring the side dishes. We have done that for years and years." The concept of *food is love* has perhaps evolved from breast-feeding. What is it about human nature that makes mothers and grandmothers want to smother their families with food? In some families, a gathering is an opportunity to cook the latest decadent recipe or show off their culinary skills. However, it is never too late to change traditions and take your family a new dish that has reduced calories. Think how much they will respect you for watching your weight and getting healthier. Maybe they will join you on the journey.

"This stuff is on my diet, maybe not this much, but at least it is fat-free." Just because it may be fat-free doesn't mean it is calorie-free, salt-free, or carb-free. And it doesn't mean you can eat two or three times as much of it because it is fat-free. The book *Eat This, Not That* exposes the misconceptions we have around restaurant foods that sound healthy but aren't. Many are two to three times the correct portion size and have three to five times the daily requirements for fat or sodium. Large restaurants are now required to post the nutritional information about their offerings. You will be able to make intelligent choices and maintain your nutritional program without being surprised. Let me just say that the author of this book does not eat at any of the nationally known fast-food restaurant chains, mostly because of the fat and sodium content of their foods.

"I am eating off program (Campbell's soup) because I am sick." We may be at our most vunerable and our guard is most down when we are not feeling well. Reverting to comfort food that produces that warm and fuzzy memory from our youth when mom's chicken soup, a piece of toast or a glass of ginger ale would cure almost any tummy upset may seem natural. Or it may just seem easier to grab that salty soup full of carbs, but it can also cause a big setback in your diet. Use the lack of appetite to your advantage.

TIP: At least try the lower-sodium and low-fat soups and the calorie-free beverages to save some calories. Add diet protein soups to low-fat chicken or beef broth and then add bits of chicken or turkey and a few veggies. Hot teas and diet hot chocolates will help.

"I missed lunch today, so I am eating more now," or "I am eating more now, but I'll make it up by working out later." Really? Few people can really do this, but the 33 percent of Americans who are *not* considered to be overweight have found a way to eat sensibly and exercise regularly. Have you? The early morning news comes on at 4:30 a.m. for a reason. Someone is watching while on an exercise bike or treadmill. Putting in that extra effort is what some people have to do to get the body they want. The benefits are supposed to be a healthier, longer life. How vigilant do you have to be? Very! As discussed earlier, just 100 extra calories a day can put 10 pounds on you over a year. According to the Centers of Disease Control and Prevention (CDC), the average American consumes an extra 125 calories at every meal. That average person burns somewhere around 125 to 150 calories an hour working out on a treadmill at a modest pace. Is it any wonder why just working out for an hour doesn't seem to be enough? Do you have five or six hours extra on the weekend to make up for all the extra bites and desserts you had during the week? As we age, it becomes even tougher to get the extra weight off. Find a routine that works for you and find ways of making it fun so that you will stick to it. Maintaining your ideal weight will then be much easier and may even be something you look forward to doing.

The foods you are addicted to are the ones you consciously or unconsciously believe will make you feel better. Once you have made the bad choice to eat it, you may even perpetuate the addiction when guilt takes over, and you may even eat more. Will that fix the problem at hand? Probably not. It is important to find a nonfood-related way to change your mood. This is where hobbies can come in or some activity you love to do when you have the time to do it. Exercise when the desire for food hits, and you should feel better for not giving into the addiction. For some, simply writing down the things you are thankful for in your life or journaling in some other manner is enough to get your mind off of food.

TIP: Joining a support group is a good idea, even after you finish maintenance on a nutritional plan. One of our favorites is Overeaters Anonymous (http://www.oa.org).

The weight you are trying to get rid of didn't come overnight and won't disappear overnight either. The main two reasons people fail at dieting are lack of focus and failure to be prepared. Stay committed no matter what life throws your way and nothing will stop you!

What are your excuses?

_____

_____

_____

_____

_____

_____

_____

_____

What should you do instead?

_____

_____

_____

_____

_____

NOTES:_____

14 ANGER

Do you think you can control your rage just by stuffing it inside? Do you try to keep it inside so no one can see your inner rage and how hurt you really are? Can that affect weight loss? Absolutely! Most people tend to stuff themselves with food when they stuff their rage. To make things worse, when you are angry, your body produces more cortisol and that makes you store more fat.

First of all, there is no one on the planet who never gets angry; we all do at one point or another. In most cases, we feel anger when we perceive something as being unfair for us or a close loved one. Beyond our loved ones, we can have a fairly thick skin to the rock and roll of life; but if one of our children is treated unfairly, watch out.

Dealing with anger in a healthy way is not easy. The sooner you discharge it, the sooner you'll get past the anger. We tend to model behavior that we were brought up observing. Holding it in and then overindulging to get over it becomes a common response. You are medicating your pain with some habitual or addictive behavior because you don't know how to get rid of it in a healthy manner. Hold it in deep and long enough and it can actually suppress your immune system and cause physical and mental problems.

Examine how you deal with it. Do you deal with anger in a healthy way? Is food involved in your efforts to relieve your stress? When you are in a situation that can induce anger, step back to look at the situation from a different point of view. When enraged, stepping back is difficult to say the least. The Peace Education Foundation has printed some Rules for Fighting Fair that can give you a good starting point.

1) Identify the problem.
2) Focus on the problem.
3) Attack the problem, not the person.
4) Listen with an open mind.
5) Treat the other person's feelings with respect.
6) Take responsibility for your actions.

Numbers one, two and three are pretty easy to see and to follow, but number four is one of the toughest things in the world to do while in the heat of an argument. Age and experience help, but only to a certain degree. Using the Rules for Fighting Fair above, your conversation with someone you are angry with should not be bawling them out in a one-sided conversation; it should be more engaging like this:

"I really feel *an emotion* when you *do this* because it makes me *feel or do this*. What I need *you to do or say or be is this*."

When you present your case to someone like this, you are not attacking them personally, just the situation. You are being assertive without being controlling. But you are controlling your anger!

Life teaches us that there are always two sides to every situation and maybe more. You must treat other people's feelings with respect. Why? Because they are allowed to have them just like you are, and they don't necessarily have to match. Take responsibility for your actions, the grown-up thing to do, because you are in control of how you respond to others, regardless of what they say or do.

The stakes get higher when what the Peace Education Foundation calls "fouls" come into play: name calling, blaming, sneering, and not listening. Any of those sound familiar? How about "getting even"? Ever bring up the past in the heat of battle? How fair is that? When will you ever forgive it? Threats, hitting, pushing, making excuses, and not taking responsibility for your

actions are all unhealthy methods of dealing with your anger.
Get in touch with how you deal with your anger. Here are some
questions to ask yourself:

1) How much do you take before your fuse flares?
2) What is the worst thing that has happened to you in the
   past because of your anger?
3) Do you feel it's OK for others to have that emotion, but
   not you?
4) Do you have to defuse arguments around you and always
   be the peacemaker?
5) Do you hold grudges?
6) Do you know when you are "hungry" versus "hangry?"
7) How much do you take before your fuse flares?
8) What is the worst thing that has happened to you because
   of your anger?
9) Do you feel it is OK for others to have that emotion, but
   not you?
10) Do you have to defuse arguments around you and always
    be the peacemaker?

Remember, there is no such thing as *never* getting angry, but
some people rarely show it. They may stuff their anger and eat
because of that. On the other hand, some people get very
embarrassed at their displays of anger and eat because of that. Road
rage is anger. Throwing things, swearing, and slamming doors can
be displays of anger. You can break physical objects and then break
your heart. How much can you take before anger turns to rage?

Again, the key is to increase your emotional tolerance and not
let whatever it is bothering you get to you. It does and will take
practice, but with positive reinforcement conditioning, you can
manage your anger. You have to find another outlet for it other
than eating. It can be exercise, talking it out, therapy, or other
healthy outlets.

If you go through life seeking revenge, getting even, or holding
grudges, the rage can build to dangerous levels. Do you have that
"I'll get you, my pretty" mentality? Do you have constructive
outlets for negative emotional energy? Constructive methods for
disposing of the negative, angry energy will go a long way in
helping you understand what makes you happy as well. Perspective
is the key. Also, a faith-based system can provide a good

foundation in dealing with the unfairness of life when you know beyond a shadow of a doubt that there is a grand plan for your life. Find inspiration in your faith and belief system to calm yourself.

This poem, "Anyway," can help you gain perspective when you feel hurt or angry. The poem is attributed to Mother Teresa and part of it is purportedly inscribed in one her children's homes in Calcutta. According to a March 8, 2002 *New York Times* article by David D. Kirkpatrick, it was originally written by Kent M. Keith.

People are often unreasonable, illogical, and self-centered;
forgive them anyway.
If you are kind, people may accuse you of selfish, ulterior motives;
be kind anyway.
If you are successful, you will win some false friends and true friends;
succeed anyway.
If you are honest and frank, people may cheat you;
be honest and frank anyway.
What you spend years building, someone could destroy overnight;
build anyway.
If you find serenity and happiness, they may be jealous;
be happy anyway.
The good you do today, people will often forget about tomorrow;
do good anyway.
Give the world the best you've got anyway.
You see, in the final analysis, it is between you and God;
it was never between you and them anyway.

The higher road is often the one less traveled, but it gains the most respect. It is character building and will improve your self-esteem, for there is never a wrong time to do the right thing. Over the long haul, it will help keep you on the right self-improvement track to becoming happy with yourself.

Find the things that have been eating you, and deal with them. Build on them and make them successes instead of bringing up the past and falling back. The past is past, and you can do nothing about it. For example, you may be angry you lost your job, but you might start your own business that becomes wildly successful; or you may be angry that you got ill and gained weight, but in the end, you may end up healthier than you ever were. The future will manifest from your positive aspirations and might turn out they exact way you have planned it. That is OK because as one of our affirmations (from chapter eighteen) says, "Everything turns out exquisitely better than I could have planned it." Live and make the most out of today because that is all we truly have; and just maybe that is why we call it "the present": because that is what we have been given.

Answer the questions on page 127:

NOTES:_____

_____

_____

_____

_____

_____

_____

_____

_____

_____

_____

_____

_____

_____

_____

_____

_____

_____

_____

_____

_____

_____

_____

_____

15 GRIEF AND LOSS

Grief and loss of a loved one is perhaps the one emotion where other people most often feel compelled to bring food to comfort you. As soon as there is a death in the community, all the neighbors descend on the grieving family with gifts of casseroles, desserts, and enough other foods to feed an army. While you may not feel like overindulging at first, in the weeks and months to come, food becomes your comfort as you grieve the loss of the family member.

However, grief and loss do not necessarily imply the death of a loved one. You can grieve the loss of a job or the loss of a marriage, for instance, and still have the same feelings of loss and still use food for comfort. Some people even pig out if they lose a prized possession, like a laptop, or if they total their car. These things can be replaced, but you still have feelings of grief. It is harder for some people than others. Think about how you react with eating to different people and things you have lost in your life.

There are no guarantees in life. We get caught up in all kinds of distraction, and then life shocks us back to this basic reality from time to time. You may have lots of years left or you may only have five minutes. You may have years left with a loved one or mere

131

moments. Your home, your job, your health—all are subject to change. Would you live your life differently if you only had five minutes or five days left? Sure you would. Have you ever wished you had told someone you loved them before they died? We find out what is really important by having the things and the people we hold most dear taken away. A family member dies unexpectedly, and we realize how little time we spent with them. All of a sudden, we realize how important family is. An old rabbi once said that the question of why God has taken our loved ones will never be answered until we get to ask Him ourselves. Until then, our question for ourselves should be, "What's next?"

Change is about the only thing that doesn't change. Everything is in a constant state of evolution, and so are we. We have the ability to adapt to new circumstances. Time seems to last forever for a child, but for a 70-year old, ten years pass in a snap of the finger. Time is matter of perspective and how much you can squeeze into a day.

One day, the sun will not come up. Scientists aren't sure about our local yellow star, but if it acts like the other medium-sized yellow stars we can observe, it will collapse and go supernova inside of 20 billion years or so, and it will vaporize our tiny blue-green planet when it does. Until then, be thankful you have another day above ground because it doesn't have to be that way.

One thing is for certain—all of our relationships will come to an end someday. The *when* may not be up to us; sometimes it is, and sometimes it isn't. After that? Not all of the 7 billion people on Earth believe in an afterlife; but when you do, it sure is easier to accept and grieve for the death of loved ones. What you believe is up to you; but I believe if you are depressed or struggling with the loss of a loved one, you should certainly investigate religion as a means of giving purpose and meaning to life.

If you have trouble appreciating your life, just ask someone who has had a brief brush with death, and they will all say they are thankful for today and thankful to be breathing. They are grateful and excited about life despite anything that happens. Their experiences with pain and the loss of health also help them learn to process grief during other hard times.

Indeed, Lee McCaskill, the author of the first part of this book, had a miraculous healing and lives with this kind of life of gratitude. She was very ill, first with mixed connective tissue disease

(MCTD) and gained over 100 pounds in four months. She lay in bed during her illness, unable to move, praying for God to help her find a way out of her fat body. Physicians at Duke University told her that MCTD was rare and that she was allergic to the few medications to relieve the symptoms—and there was no cure. They pretty much gave up on her and told her to go home and try to enjoy the rest of her life. Determined to get well, she got rid of household chemicals, got rid of every food in a can or a box, and she started taking herbs and vitamins. She began a series of diet plans, trying to find one that worked for her, and she prayed, really prayed, that God would help her find a way out of her fat body. Some deals were made. She felt so strongly about it that she promised if she found a way, she would help everyone else!

Just as Lee thought she was almost well from one illness, another struck—every lymph gland on her body enlarged almost overnight. She was diagnosed with lymphoma after a positive biopsy. Then, three days before surgery, she had an angel vision and was miraculously cured of lymphoma! She felt God had healed her for the mission she prayed about, but what was she thinking—she had no money and no weight loss plan. Through a long series of coincidences, otherwise known as God's plan for her, money came from nowhere and her aunt formulated a weight loss plan for her, without Lee even asking for it. She lost an amazing 93 pounds between the previous diets she had done and the one her aunt formulated. Within two years, Lee had four thriving weight loss clinics. Several years later, she added a network of out-of-town consultants to her team to counsel clients all over the U.S. And now you are reading this book! She has been an inspiration to thousands of people because of her faith and a promise she made to God in the depths of her worst despair.

Lee believes she was able to handle the deaths of both of her parents much more easily because of seeing the angel. She says she went from hoping with faith to knowing with intimate knowledge that another realm exists. Maybe it is a shame that we don't all get that experience, but we can read about it.

Heaven Is for Real is a best-selling book by Todd Burpo that tells the story of his then 4-year-old son's near-death experience. His son's spontaneous, off-the-cuff descriptions of where he went, what he did, and who he was with are not seasoned with predispositions, but came from the pure angelic mind of a young uncluttered soul. His account is a refreshing and affirming story that reminds us of the countless other stories of those who have been clinically deceased and returned with a whole new attitude on this life. There have been too many occurrences to discount their possibility, and yet there are never enough to dispel the skeptics. Perhaps we would be wise not to bet against it.

Terry Kellogg and Marvel Harrison say in their book, *Finding Balance,* that since we all will face losses in life, it makes sense that all of us will accept and grieve those losses differently. We will each grieve in our own way and some will come to acceptance faster than others. They describe the grieving process as a process of saying good-bye and a pathway to connecting to the new unknown that lies ahead. The process includes feelings we all experience after a death of a loved one: denial, fear, bargaining, depression, sadness, and acceptance. Most all of us go through these six phases of grief, but some go through them faster than others do. It is surely a time to look within ourselves and find out who we really are and what we hold valuable.

Unfortunately, along the way we have learned some very unhealthy ways to grieve our losses that set us up for depression, emptiness, guilt, and shame. Here are the lessons we have learned.

1) **Don't feel. Stuff your pain; it really doesn't hurt that bad, and many others have it way worse than you have.** Stuffing your feelings is not a healthy thing to do, and it can have horrific consequences in your daily life. Feelings take energy and need to be expressed, not bottled up. TIP: A website created for families dealing with grief, www.hellogrief.org, says "With every story you tell, you heal; and with every story you hear, you heal as well." Talking about what you are feeling is healing, and hearing how others have dealt with similar circumstances is helpful in dealing with what is going on inside you as well.

2) **Replace the loss immediately.** Wanting something to take away the feeling of emptiness you are experiencing is a common but unhealthy occurrence. How many people do you know that will replace a pet within days or weeks? Or replace even a husband or wife? It is, unfortunately, a form of denial. TIP: Concentrate after the death of a loved one on a memorial garden, scholarship, or something in their honor, but don't replace the relationship immediately.

3) **Grieve alone.** There's no reason to bring down everyone else around you with your problems. Do you feel like you may make them unhappy just because you might be? Do you think they don't need to see you in pain and upset? That's rubbish. Your friends will be there for you just like you will be there for them, because that's what friends do. Acquaintances may not, but friends will. **TIP:** Consider joining a grief support group moderated by a professional counselor. You will meet people going through the same thing you are and will truly understand.

4) **Time will heal the loss, but don't take too much time.** Remember, we will all grieve in our way, at our own pace; but in a place of employment, time off is usually only three days. Is that long enough to get over it? For some, yes; but if it was a close loved one, probably not. Many take this time for self-introspection and as a time to make changes because the reality of how short life is really comes home. **TIP:** Don't assume because you are over someone's death that everyone else around you is and vice versa.

5) **Watch how others handle the loss.** We model our expected behavior by observing our parents, older siblings, and others we admire. However, what feels right for them may not feel right for us. We learn by trying different coping mechanisms until one feels right for us. Some cultures will celebrate the recently departed with a huge celebration. Others will hardly mention it, and treat it like a speed bump on a long highway. You have to find a way within yourself to cope. **TIP:** Don't let others tell you how to handle your grief. For example, one person may want to clean out a deceased person's closets immediately and another may want to wait a year or so; when to clean them out should not be dictated by well-meaning friends. It has to be done when *you* are ready.

Getting caught up in trying to find out the *why* only sets us up for disappointment, sadness, and depression. As the old rabbi once said, "We will never know why." We cannot change the past. Hopefully, we learn from it and do not repeat the mistakes. Our job is to be ready when our Maker comes calling. Are you? Do you live each day like it's "the present" we have been given to enjoy?

Do you make the world a better place for you being in it each and every day?

This poem is called "After a While" by Veronica Shoffstall. It is available at http://www.scribd.com/doc/3946382/After-a-While-Veronica-A-Shoffstall#force_seo.

After awhile you learn the subtle difference
between holding a hand and chaining a soul.
And you learn that love doesn't mean leaning
and company doesn't always mean security.
And you begin to learn
That kisses aren't contracts
And presents aren't promises
And you begin to accept your defeats
With you head up and your eyes ahead
With the grace of a woman
Not the unresolved grief of a child

And you learn
To build all your roads on today
Because tomorrow's ground is
Too uncertain for plans
And futures have a way
Of falling down in mid flight
After a while, you learn
That even sunshine burns if you get too much
So you plant your own garden
And decorate your own soul
Instead of waiting
For someone to bring you flowers
And you learn
That you really can endure
That you really are strong
And you really do have worth
And you learn and you learn.
With every good bye you learn.

What did you get out of this poem?_____

_____

16 STRESS AND RELAXATION

Don't worry, be happy—and relaxed. No doubt about it, stress is probably sabotaging your dieting success. According to a Centers for Disease Control and Prevention report, an overwhelming percentage of the people who are 30 pounds or more overweight report that stress was the number one reason for their overeating. What signs do you look for that will tell you that the stress of daily life is getting to you? Not sleeping well? Indigestion? A nervous tic? Depression or irritability? Drinking or smoking more? Eating ice cream right out of the container in the middle of the night? Do you find yourself lashing out and being a bit insubordinate? You might even start cocooning, using the silent treatment, or internalizing everything. Reading can be an escape to avoid having to talk about what is bothering you. Maybe you even pick on someone weaker than you are. Some people will even get psychosomatic diseases to avoid stress, physically making themselves ill to avoid the situation.

Changing your mood with food is a conditioned response we learn from birth. Do you find yourself gravitating to a specific comfort food to make yourself feel better when you're upset or feel like the world is closing in on you? Awareness is half the battle. Ignorance is bliss. If you have no idea why you are eating a particular comfort food, that's OK, but you may want to investigate to improve your future. For instance, one of our clients figured out that her ice cream addiction came from her early childhood, when the only time that her dad paid her any attention was when they shared ice cream together. Another client figured out that his addiction to bread came from his deep love for his German grandmother's homemade bread.

There are five ways we normally respond to stress: fighting, fleeing, freezing, coping, and preventative health care. The changes your body will make to deal with stress, perceived or real, are quite amazing. They have been in development for thousands of years as humans found a way to survive in a hostile world. The first two responses, the fight or flight response, is a defense mechanism man has had since he lived in a cave. The fight response can be verbal, rebellion, a passive-aggressive silent treatment, sabotage, or it can be as simple as the displacement, kick-the-cat syndrome. Displacement is where Dad is upset about not getting a raise at work, so he comes home and yells at his wife for no reason, and then his wife takes it out on her daughter by telling her she can't go out on a date, and the daughter takes it out on her little brother by telling him he can no longer use her computer, and the brother kicks the cat. The cat would have never gotten kicked if all that displacement had not happened!

The fleeing response to stress is a little trickier because we cannot always physically leave a situation. So we flee in other ways: denial (acting as though there is no stress), suppression (pretending it doesn't hurt), fantasizing, giving up emotionally, regressing, getting sick or having an accident, turning to an addiction such as drugs, alcohol, sex or overeating.

The third response to stress is freezing, and that rarely lasts very long because of our jobs or other responsibilities. Freezing just means we become indecisive or procrastinate, putting off a response until later. By then we may have of the first two responses—fight or flight—or have figured out a way to do the next two, coping or getting stronger and dealing with the situation. A coping response can involve either mental techniques (like imagery, music, or affirmations) or physical techniques (like exercise, breathing techniques, massage, or a warm bath). As a last resort, the physical answer may be medication.

In the long run, preventative health care is the key to reducing the stress and counteracting the effects of stressors you can't eliminate. You get stronger. You work in a job you enjoy, have fun in your life, and adhere to a faith that sustains you. You work on building balance in your life using techniques like those shown here and taking care of yourself mentally and physically. And you can take herbal supplements, like resveratrol or raspberry ketone, to keep your body from storing fat when it is under stress because of the extra cortisol released. (Both of those can be ordered at our website http://www.bestdietsource.com.) Also, having some good, constructive methods for dealing with stress in your life is a must.

Here are some better coping techniques to help you respond to stress:

1) **Get organized:** When you organize the twenty-four hours you have in a day, you will find extra time to do things after sleeping and taking care of your obligations. Be realistic and estimate how much of your time it will take to accomplish your tasks, sleeping, eating, etc. Plot it out for a week, and don't forget to leave some time to recharge your batteries. Plan only 75 percent of your day so that you can allow for the unexpected things that will come up. Make room for Murphy's Law, and you will reduce the chaos that can cause unnecessary stress. If Murphy doesn't show up, the extra time will be for you!

TIP: This is Lee's favorite site for everything from cleaning house to office organization: http://www.flylady.net/

2) **Turn off the news:** Set your Internet news service for only the subjects that you want to know about. The selling of the news is stressful in itself. All of the teases and "expert" opinions that make you feel like the world is on the edge of total doom are just designed to keep you tuned in until we get back from a commercial break. Don't become addicted to the news.

TIP: Read all your news condensed in one place to save time: https://www.reddit.com/.

3) **Reward your good behavior:** Divide your big goals to a series of smaller goals that fit a reasonable timeline. Find nonfood-related ways to celebrate the successes while on your journey. Cut out pictures of what you want, and make a vision board with them the old-fashioned, cut-and-paste way. Place it in a very conspicuous place to remind

yourself of why you are working so hard. It is too easy to change your mind and get discouraged when your objectives are not clear. Put things on it that make you happy at the very thought of them. Be specific and don't short-change yourself. Dream big—you deserve it. Pat yourself on the back if no one else will.

TIP: Chapter eighteen "How to Do Affirmations" contains links for making mind movies about your goals and how to use Jack Canfield's vision boards.

"No matter who you are, no matter what you did, no matter where you've come from, you can always become a better version of yourself." —Madonna

4) **Find something you *love* to do:** Whatever that may be, it should get you to forget about all of your problems and worries. Creative endeavors are great ways to keep the mind engaged. Watersports, tennis, racquetball, biking, and other sports can be exercise as well as forms of unwinding. Playing a musical instrument, painting, doing needlepoint, journaling, reading, or learning a new skill are all great activities for unwinding, too. Volunteer your time to a charity or join organizations that do positive things in your local community. When you are helping others with their problems, you tend to forget your own. Did you know that gardening is the number one relaxing activity practiced in America? A whopping 75 percent of all Americans do their gardening on anything from a farm to an acre to an apartment balcony. If not the thrill of seeing something you planted grow, pulling a few weeds may just make you feel better. If you can figure out a way to get paid for gardening or something else you love to do, you win big time.

TIP: This claims to be the biggest list of hobbies that exists, so surely you will find something interesting to get involved in: http://www.stormthecastle.com/the-list-of-hobbies.htm.

5) **Music soothes the savage beast:** Listening to a CD by your favorite group is a sixty-minute great escape. The mind can hold the words to over 2,000 songs, so you don't want to play songs with words in them and end up playing

Name That Tune. Try soothing instrumental music like jazz or classical music that doesn't have lyrics when you are trying to relax.

TIP: To find music with only instrumentals, search the word *instrumentals* in the search bar. You can listen to them on your computer and then download them to your Spotify account for free: http://www.last.fm/music.

6) **Deep diaphragmatic breathing:** We tend to forget to breathe when we are stressed out. Your breathing becomes shortened, robbing your brain of oxygen just when you need it to work at an optimal level. Getting fresh air to the bottom of our lungs requires our diaphragm to flex fully. Deep breathing can also accelerate our metabolism up to 20 percent. Earlier in the book, Lee described how to properly do these deep-breathing exercises. Get a few deep ones in whenever you fell stressed. Do ten when you first wake up, and ten when you are ready to fall asleep. Do a few to step back from the edge for a few seconds. Lee recommends doing them at every stoplight and during every TV commercial. Co-workers go out for a smoke break? You deserve a stress break, don't you? When you are in the bathroom at work, close the door and do breathing exercises, too. In proper diaphragmatic breathing, the belly button should rise higher than the chest. Inhaling and exhaling should last three to four seconds. Breathe in through the nose, allowing the air to be gently warmed, and breathe out slowly by mouth, releasing the stress. The benefits certainly outweigh the costs. It's free and can help you lose weight faster, so why wouldn't you do this?

TIP: We recommend Jill Johnson's Oxycise videos; not only do they have breathing exercises, they also have mild workouts on them that any age can do. The site has plenty of info but you have to order the videos and they are well-worth the money: http://www.oxycise.com/whatis.htm .

7) **Think:** The old trick of counting to ten can give you a few moments to think about what you are going to say and how someone might take it. Is it positive and helpful, or

destructive and negative? It will help keep you from over-reacting and saying something you really didn't mean to say in the heat of battle. If someone says something that hurts you or your feelings, rather than lashing out at them, ask them right then if that was their intention. Calmly ask them to please not do that again. Keeping a positive attitude is just not a cliché. It makes your world a better place to be and, according to the Mayo Clinic, it can make you healthier as well.

TIP: Look at this out-of-the-box, new way Indian doctors are suggesting to patients to control their anger by adding humor to the old trick of counting to ten. It works; try it! http://doctor.ndtv.com/photodetail/ndtv/id/7706/10_Tips_on_Anger_Management.html.

8) **Exercise:** A short walk around the block or a grueling forty-five-minute aerobic workout will help get your mind off what's stressing you and make you feel better. Your body will release endorphins and serotonin that will change your mood. Walking is much better for you than eating, for sure. Even stretching for fifteen to twenty minutes will help get the blood circulating. Anybody can stretch. Instead of thinking about snacking during commercial breaks, you could do arm exercises with a one- or two-pound weight. Don't have any? A 16-ounce can of vegetables weighs one pound! Get inventive: Leg lifts are easy, so are stomach crunches. Just starting is the key. Work your way up from a can of veggies to a gallon jug of water that weighs 8 pounds when full, and half-full is about 4 pounds. You will be able to track your progress and meet small goals that will turn into big major changes. Do what you can do, and don't think about what you can't. You will feel better about yourself.

TIP: Our website has a virtual gym on the site at http://bestdietsource.gostorego.com/gym.html that you can use to find individual exercises, do an at-home program with a virtual trainer, order equipment, hire a trainer near you, or find the nearest gym. Check it out!

9) **Get mentally stronger and increase your willpower:** Exercise your mind with games, puzzles, creative thought, meditation, self-improvement courses, or reading—even watching *Jeopardy* can help keep your mind sharp. Challenge yourself to master things that don't come easy. Getting mentally stronger occurs when you gain the confidence that comes with trusting yourself to do what you have said you were going to do. Developing an unshakable self-confidence lets you know there isn't anything you can't do if you really focus and put your mind to it. Sometimes you might have to take it minute by minute to get through the threat to your commitment. Temptations will be everywhere, and you have to resist them no matter what they are and how tempting they might be. At times, you will be challenged with every breath you take. Keep the promise you made to yourself no matter what life throws at you, and you will be able to achieve anything you want to do.

TIP: Read *The Seat of the Soul* by Gary Zukav. Oprah Winfrey says it is the best book she has ever read other than the Bible. It will change the way you see the world, interact with other people, and help you better understand your own actions and motivations. Gary Zukav believes we have evolved from a species that competes for energy from the world and its beings and understands power as the ability to manipulate and control (external power) into a species that is beginning to cooperate and share energy and understand power as the alignment of the personality with the soul (authentic power).

10) **A hot tub or spa visit can do magic:** The Romans may have invented the hot bath, but Mr. Jacuzzi may have perfected it. There is nothing like a hot bubble tub to take your troubles to another place far, far away. Fifteen minutes later, you're refreshed and relaxed—ahhhhhhhh. Tubs come in all sizes from a cozy two-person spa up to a twelve-person giant model. There is even an inflatable hot tub that can be set up indoors. A trip to a spa is a great reward while on your weight reduction journey. Every minor goal along the way, be it 10, 15, or 25 pounds, deserves a half day or so of pampering. A massage, mud

bath, pedicure, and facial are certainly things to look forward to and will help keep you on track.

TIP: If you are on a budget, try some at-home spa treatments. Our favorites online sites for ideas are:

    a. http://www.glamour.com/lipstick/2008/11/13-diy-at-home-spa-tricks/13

    b. http://www.thedatingdivas.com/you-me/lookin-good-for-your-spouse/25-relaxing-diy-spa-night-ideas/

    c. And then one with everything you can imagine: http://www.spaindex.com/recipes/

    d. If you like body wraps, not only are they relaxing, here is one that will help you lose 3-4 pounds per wrap and 7-20 inches each time because it has neem oil in it that melts fat! http://tropicalspawraps.com/

11) **Change the lighting:** Fluorescent bulbs in the office can cause stress, so try adding an incandescent lamp to more closely mimic outdoor light. It will help regulate your natural biorhythms, decrease mood swings and depression, and combat Seasonal Affective Disorder (SAD). Candlelight is not only more romantic in your bedroom at night, it also sends a message to the brain to release melatonin. That will help you get a better night's sleep and keep stress levels at a minimum. Your immune system will thank you as well.

 TIP: Here is a link to many different kinds of lamps, all for SAD: http://www.fullspectrumsolutions.com/light_therapy_13_ct.htm

12) **Display your best moments:** Looking at pictures of your successes can help reset your brain so that anticipating the best outcomes becomes the expected, not the exception. Try to find images of three of your best days so you can remember how you felt. It might be dancing at your wedding, winning a sporting event, or receiving an award

of some kind. Staring at them for at least ten seconds a day can help lower muscle tension, lower your heart rate, and refuel your desire to experience that great feeling again. **TIP:** These images can be the screensaver on your computer so that you see them when you turn on your computer each day.

13) **Practice an attitude of gratitude:** An attitude of gratitude goes a long way in handling the stresses of daily life in our fast-paced world. Don't hold back on compliments when someone deserves it, and don't feel like you have to receive one in return. But practice being an excellent receiver when you do get a compliment and be sincerely gracious.
TIP: Visit a place that claims to be the happiest place on the internet: http://www.gratitudelog.com/. Also, take the challenge at :http://www.30daygratitudechallenge.com/ and let us know what happens when you participate!

14) **Practice affirmations:** You might try repeating an affirmation or two when you start feeling a bit anxious in order to help you calm down. Affirmations cement a belief in your head and make you stronger. A favorite that works time and time again is, "Everything happens exquisitely better than I could have possibly planned." (See chapter eighteen "How to Do Affirmations".) **TIP:** For affirmations that are already written (you can pick your choice of music to go with them), visit:

- http://www.orindaben.com/pages/rooms/affirmat ions_room - null
- http://www.poweraffirmations.com/?page_id=195 0

15) **Meditate:** Guided imagery in a sea of positivity eases tension and anxiety. It can help you gain clarity, maintain focus, and provide the sequencing needed for whatever tasks may be. There are many methods that can get to a space where you can stop your internal dialogue and just be. Allow your thoughts to just flow without direction. This process will take a lot of practice in the beginning, but

it will take just a few minutes once you are good at it. Find a comfortable chair or lie down in a quiet place. Turn the TV off and find some soothing background noise, like the ocean, a quiet rhythmic fan, sounds of nature, or something without words. Take in ten deep breaths slowly, to a count of three or four. Exhale just as slowly, telling yourself to release the stresses of the day and relax. Next, relax with your toes and work your way up your body, all the way to the top of your head. The sequence should be future, present, and past. As you work your way up, in your head, it will sound something like this: "My toes are going to relax...my toes are relaxing...my toes are now very relaxed...the bottoms of my feet are going to relax..." And so on. Allow at least a minute for each body part. Take as much time as necessary. If your back or hips need more time, take it. The more stressed you are, the more detailed the journey. When you get to the top, tell your body it is now completely relaxed and calm. You may feel the sensations of floating. Now stop talking and just "be". Stay in that space as long as you can—at least ten to fifteen minutes, if possible. This seems like it would be very easy to do, but it's not. It will take lots and lots of practice to stay in the zone for fifteen minutes, maybe even a lifetime.

This is also a great technique for falling asleep. It is certainly relaxing and is a must-have technique for overachievers. Some claim it is as good as a two- to three-hour nap for revitalizing your energy and clearing your head. Thomas Edison used this method, as have a number of other great thinkers.

TIP: Here are links to two teachers of meditation that Oprah Winfrey recommends:

- http://www.learnoutloud.com/Free-Audio-Video/Self-Development/Prayer-and-Meditation/21Day-Meditation-Challenge/46927
- http://www.eomega.org/workshops/teachers/panache-desai

Managing your stress will be key to your maintaining balance in your life as you strive to be as successful as you can be. Will there be challenges? Absolutely. Will you reframe every threat into a challenge and make the best of it? You hope so. Do you have to be perfect? No, you don't. Accept the fact that no one is perfect, and just strive to be magnificent!

"Nothing gives one person so much advantage over another as to remain cool and unruffled under all circumstances." —Thomas Jefferson

Did you go to any of the links listed? (It may be easier from the e-book available online) If so, what helped you the most?

_____

_____

_____

_____

_____

_____

_____

_____

_____

Would you recommend any of these or this book to friends and why?

_____

_____

_____

_____

_____

_____

_____

Nancy Lee McCaskill & Michael Vernon

NOTES:_____

_____

_____

_____

_____

_____

_____

_____

_____

_____

_____

_____

_____

_____

_____

_____

_____

_____

_____

_____

_____

_____

17 HOW TO HAVE UNSHAKABLE SELF-ESTEEM

"You deserve to be happy, you deserve to be joyful, and you deserve to be celebrated. But, in order to do that you must first fall madly in love with yourself...no matter what."—Lisa Nichols, author of *No Matter What!*

You can't *pretend* to have self-esteem, and you can't buy it at a store. Once you have dealt with, maybe even mastered, all of the things mentioned in this book you may have acquired a great deal of self-esteem. But is it unshakable? No matter what life throws your way, you are ready to handle it with grace: cool, calm, and collected?

When I ask students what self-esteem is, I get answers like, "It is how you feel about yourself," or "It is how others perceive you," but rarely do I get anything about a person's level of self-confidence. How you feel about yourself only describes a portion of self-esteem, but the confidence you have in yourself is a bigger slice of the pie.

Your level of self-esteem has an effect on your health, creativity, the quality of your relationships, your ability to handle money, and it has a big effect on your ability to actualize your full potential. It is one of the most important things to have in your life. It is a true manifestation of your inner spirit engaged in the action of your life. Therefore, it is the core of your spiritual state—much more than how you feel about yourself. It has much to do with how you handle stress and chaos as it presents itself going through daily life.

You increase your level of self-esteem through a series of self-accomplishments. You cannot pretend to have it because until you actually accomplish it there is always a slight amount of doubt that you can do it. You have to do it to get it.

To quote Terry Kellogg, "Self-esteem and self-worth develop from the inside. It is not based on things outside of yourself such as weight, clothes, material possessions, children, or whatever. It is increased when you feel comfortable within yourself in the various domains in your life, and when you do esteemable things for yourself, not necessarily what you do for others in your life. There may be areas in your life that you wish to improve upon, like your weight; however, if you base your self-worth on what you look like rather who you really are, you will go back to where you are right now."

So, who are you?

If you don't know, now is the time to find out. Read each of these questions and write down your answers to them so that you can review them later.

- Have you based your view of yourself on what other people have said?
- Have you always tried to please or serve others before serving yourself?
- Do you feel guilty when you do things for yourself when so many others are in need?
- Are you a manifestation of your environment, or do you control your own destiny?
- What do you like about yourself, and what don't you like?
- Are you willing and ready to change?
- Do you fear change?
- What else do you fear?
- How do you feel when you venture outside of your comfort zone?
- How would you like to be remembered? Have you ever thought of what you want your tombstone to read? Are you living your life that way now?
- What are your values and principles?

The answers to these questions will define who and what you are. Write down your first impulses and revisit them during your weight loss process and after you reach your goal weight. You just may surprise yourself and see yourself growing. Keeping a journal is a great method of getting in touch with your feelings to find out if you are an emotional eater and grow in awareness of why you were overeating in the first place. Awareness is half the battle.

You want to describe yourself with words like *integrity*, *character*, *honorable*, and *trustworthy*. According to Webster:

Integrity – n. 1. Firm adherence to a code or standard of values 2. The state of being unimpaired 3. The quality or condition of being undivided

Character – n. 1. The combination of emotional, intellectual, and moral qualities distinguishing one person or group from another 3. Moral or ethical strength

According to Successories, the motivational calendar and poster people:

Integrity – Have the courage in the face of adversity to travel the path of Integrity without looking back, for there is never a wrong time to do the right thing.

Character – Your true character is revealed by the clarity of your convictions. Hold strongly to your principles and refuse to follow the currents of convenience.

And one more, a bit more than 3,000 years old, coming from Heraclitus:

Integrity – *The soul is dyed the color of its thoughts. Think only of those things that can bear the full light of day. The content of your character is your choice. Day by day, what you choose, what you think, and what you do is who you become. Your Integrity is your destiny…it is the light that guides your way.*

Right now is when your self-esteem and recovery start. So what one thing do you need to do differently first so you can keep the unwanted weight off forever? Start with one change and build on that. Keep the promises you make yourself, no matter what life throws at you. It is that simple. How many times have you made a promise to yourself, only to break it a few hours or days later? Probably more times than you care to remember. Who is the easiest person to break a promise to? Yourself? Are there any consequences to breaking the promises you make yourself? Perhaps not any on the surface, other than a little delayed gratification; but that's no big deal, right? Wrong! Look in the mirror—there are the consequences. What you see is too much of you in the mirror, in spite of your good intentions. You have found a way of rationalizing. You told yourself you were not going to give in to food temptations, but you did. Perhaps you made bad decisions. Remember, your choices determine your destiny. Make better choices and don't break that promise, no matter what. Draw the line and good changes will happen.

Do you think your attitude has anything to do with this? Of course it does. Maintaining a good or positive attitude when everything seems to be falling apart around you isn't easy, but who said life was going to be easy?

"Tough times never last, but tough people do." —Dr. Robert H. Schuller

When life throws you lemons, do you make lemonade? There are countless analogies and great sayings about maintaining a positive attitude and not all are clichés. No one says it better than Charles Swindoll, a former US Marine, who founded Insight for Living in Plano, Texas, and is senior pastor at Stonebriar Community Church in Frisco, Texas. He has authored more than 70 books, and was named as one of the Top 25 preachers of the past 50 years by *Christianity Today* magazine. Swindoll says, "The longer I live, the more I realize the impact of ATTITUDE on life. ATTITUDE, to me, is more important than education, than money, than circumstances, than failure, than success, than what other people think, say, or do. It is more important than appearance, giftedness, or skill. It will make or break a company, a church, or a home. The remarkable thing is that we have a choice everyday regarding that ATTITUDE we embrace for that day. We cannot change the past…we cannot change the fact that people will act in a certain way. We cannot change the inevitable. The only thing we can do is play on the one string we have, and that is our ATTITUDE. I am convinced that the life is 10 percent what happens to me and 90 percent how I react to it. And so it is with you, we are in charge of our ATTITUDES."

That quote is the motto of the self-proclaimed number one seafood restaurant in South Carolina, Charleston's Hyman's Seafood. It is also found framed in all of Lee McCaskill's Before and After Weight Loss Clinics.

This essay, "Stream of Consciousness" by Bill Marshall, explains why positive thought is so vital.

One thing that is important to realize about thought; one thought always leads to another. It is impossible to have one thought without having another one. What does this have to do with positive and negative thinking? Everything. The thoughts usually follow one after another—usually in a similar vein, until there is some type of interruption that changes the thought pattern. Sometimes the interruption is outside of ourselves. Other times, the interruption is something we initiate when we take conscious control of our thoughts.

So, the point is this: Thoughts follow one another and eventually create a stream of thought. A stream of consciousness. The questions you have to ask is how clear or positive is your stream? If you are protecting your thoughts, consciously keeping them positive, then positive circumstances will generally flow. If you just 'go with the flow' without consciously taking control of your own mind, it is almost inevitable that a high percentage of pollution or negative thinking will find its way into your 'stream.'

So, if you want to keep your thoughts positive, it is absolutely crucial that you feed your mind success-related thoughts every day. It can come from books, audio programs, affirmations, or whatever. The more positive material you feed it, the less time your mind will wander. Eventually your mind will be so positive, there won't be any room left for negative thoughts.

You cannot afford the penalty of a single negative thought because there is no such thing as just a <u>single</u> negative thought. Resolve to take control of your mind this moment and fill your mind, and the world around you, with positive thought.

June Scobee Rodgers is the wife of former astronaut Richard Scobee, commander of the shuttle Challenger, which blew up just seventy-three seconds after liftoff. The trial and tribulations of her life can make this journey to positive thinking as simple as A-B-C! She developed a way of looking at life that got her through some of the most trying times. Growing up, she was the oldest of three children. Her mother used to take the kids on outings to cities without a plan, money, or a place to stay. Crazy? Growing up and dealing with that reality made June a tough lady. She developed a survival system to deal with her mother's instability, the death of her husband, and the shock of losing the six other brave Americans who were with her husband. Her survival system that got her through her mother's antics and the tragic death of the Challenger crew is as simple as A…B…C. Her system can help you as well to get back on track and to keep your eye on the prize when life throws you challenges. It is a great system to remember for weight loss programs.

A. **Stands for Attitude:** A positive attitude can get you though many difficult times and situations.

B. **Stands for Belief:** Do you really believe you can stick to your guns and stay on your new nutritional program, no matter what life throws you?

C. **Stands for Commitment:** How committed are you? Are you willing to do whatever it takes to reach your goal? Can you stand up to your family, your mother, your coworkers, the little devil on your shoulder that says, "Life is short, go ahead, what the heck?"

June organized the spouses of the Challenger crew to carry on the mission that founded the Challenger Center for Space Science Education. To date, there are more than 500,000 students in the Challenger Center programs each year, all as a result of her survival system. She has her Ph.D. from Texas A & M University and is author of *Silver Linings: My Life Before And After* Challenger 7.

Is it really that easy—as easy as A-B-C? It has been said that the only reason we fail at anything is lack of focus. Remember the big moments in your life, the ones where you had to push yourself to do things that were way outside your comfort zone or where you had to overcome failure. Weren't those the most satisfying? Building your self-confidence and self-esteem happens through a series of self-accomplishments. It doesn't always happen on the first try. You keep doing it, failing forward to success. Now, relate this to your own weight loss.

Earl Nightingale, a sage from the last century, known as the Dean of Personal Development, is the author of *The Strangest Secret*. Nightingale was inspired by Napoleon Hill's book, *Think and Grow Rich,* which says, "We become what we think about." Nightingale defined success as "the gradual progression towards a worthwhile goal." Notice he did not say the achievement of the goal. It is the journey. So in weight loss terms, you are a success every minute of every hour of every day that you stick to your guns and stick to the plan, regardless of the temptation or perceived hardships life presents. You will smile at yourself every time you look in the mirror, knowing you were able to keep the promise to yourself and to not give in to temptation. As your body shrinks in physical size, your self-esteem is going to grow in proportion. There isn't *anything* you can't do if you put your mind to it. Every night you can go to sleep knowing you are, indeed, a success. How can that not make you feel good about yourself?

Stop worrying about failure, and start moving toward success. Throw out every excuse. "I can't" has never done a thing, but "I'll give it a try" has moved mountains!

Speaking of mountains, have you ever heard of a man named Erik Weihenmayer? He has done some astonishing things, including climbing the tallest mountains on all seven continents. That is a feat completed by a very few and is remarkable to say the least. What makes it even more special for Erik is that he is blind. He can't see when he gets to the top of the mountain. When asked why he would do such a thing he responds, "I just wanted to show all of the disabled people out there that there isn't anything you couldn't do if you put your mind to it." He's even escorted an entire class of blind students up Mt. Rainier in Washington for the same reason. As a dieter, you need to have that same attitude.

Here is more inspiration to stick to your guns and to keep the promise you made to yourself, no matter what life throws at you. Lisa Nichols, who appeared in the book and movie *The Secret*, is known in the motivational industry as "The Breakthrough Specialist". She wrote a book called *No Matter What!: 9 Steps to Living the Life You Love,* which gives the basic steps to maintaining focus and your commitment to yourself and your promise. She recommends utilizing creative visualization to help train your subconscious to change what it focuses attention on. Remember, it is said that the only reason we fail at anything is because of lack of focus. Lisa says to get pictures of what you want in life and the body you want to have, put them all on a poster or corkboard, and put it somewhere you will see it every day to remind you of what it is you really want. Also, put a picture of yourself in the body you want on your refrigerator, the mirror in the bathroom, and in your car to remind your subconscious of the shape you want to be in. It will help you make better food choices and eventually lead you to your weight loss success. It will help you pause for just a few moments to ask yourself, "Is there a better choice?" It will do wonders for keeping you on track.

Lisa is also a coauthor of *Chicken Soup for the African American Woman's Soul* with Jack Canfield and Mark Victor Hansen and penned *Unbreakable Spirit: Rising Above the Impossible.* Her own journey from struggling as a single mom in Los Angeles to being a multimillionaire can inspire anyone to the greatness that lies inside.

TIP: Here are two resources for creative visualization: 1) Jack Canfield's vision boards complete with motivational sayings and tips: http://jackcanfield.com/products/vision-board-collection/), and 2) mind movies, like what Lee uses to create a movie using PowerPoint, or the movie creator you already have on your computer; you can use it as a screensaver, reminding you daily of your goals: http://www.mindmovies.com?a_aid=6a878fbd.

Keep the focus on your goal and be tenacious about your ability to succeed. In his book *Three Feet from Gold* (coauthored with Sharon Lechter), Greg Reid outlines a human tendency to quit just before success. Do you quit most endeavors when you are three feet from gold? If that sounds like you, perhaps you should read his book. Greg is president of the Napoleon Hill Foundation and was asked to write the follow up to *Think and Grow Rich.* He also puts on "Secret Knock" seminars all over the country helping people realize their full potential.

The subconscious can sabotage your success, so be ready. It has a need for closure. It doesn't like open-ended things because they can lead to chaos and uncertainty. If you want to *lose* weight, the subconscious wants you to find it once it's been lost. Try to find a different word to associate with getting rid of the unwanted weight so the subconscious won't have that conflict. *Dissolve, get rid of, eliminate,* or even *delete* work great. The *finding it* won't be such an association problem then. This association goes back a long way in our lives. Did you ever have to go to the lost and found to find a missing glove or hat in school? If you misplace your glasses or keys, you go through every room in the house looking high and low for the missing item. Not using the word *lose* or *lost* will stop your subconscious from needing to find something; it will increase your odds of making this weight reduction permanent. Your new lifestyle is your new way of eating and is your new nutritional program for the rest of your long, healthy, and happy life! You are on your way to unshakable self-esteem!

Here are some ways to help you build your self-esteem

- Let yourself be yourself.
- Give yourself permission to try out different selves, but don't command yourself to make major changes to your true self.
- Allow yourself to *have* and *express* feelings. (You have to feel the lows to enjoy the highs.)
- Allow yourself to move, grow, change—and succeed! Always be seeking improvement and learning new things.
- Allow yourself to have personal space. Take some personal time and make dates with yourself. Enjoy your company. After all, if you think about it, no one else is as well in tune into *your* wants, needs, and desires and interests as *you* are.
- Give your support to others and learn to accept theirs in return.
- Set realistic expectations for yourself. Break big goals down into bite-sized pieces.
- Make sensuality a high priority. Re-stimulating your tactile sensitivity can add a new dimension to your life experience.
- Try new things and allow yourself to make mistakes.
- Express valid personal wants and needs.
- Take responsibility for your thoughts, feelings, and ideas.
- Work on communication skills. Keep the lines of communication open.
- Learn to read other people and become aware of yourself as well.
- Start receiving pleasure as well as giving it.
- Accept your body the way it is. It is the first step in changing it.
- Become aware of your body image. Visualize what you look like walking into a room.
- Listen to what you sound like.
- Learn to say "no" without feeling guilty.
- Take time each day to relax. Practice meditation or deep breathing exercises. This is a great stress reliever.

- Become aware of the things that reinforce you and use them.
- Listen to your body. It will tell you all kinds of things—like when you are hungry, when you are full, when you are tired, when you need to do something active.
- Allow yourself to fantasize. Be careful what you *act* on. If you fantasize that you can do something you felt was impossible, it just may come to pass!
- Visualize yourself with high self-esteem. Hear yourself and feel yourself in successful situations.
- Look *up*. The old saying, "Things are looking up," actually has some truth to it. Your posture can make you feel better and cause you to be perceived that you are feeling better than you actually are.
- Make a list of things you really like about yourself or things you do well. Ask others to make the same kinds of lists for you.
- Catch yourself doing things right and pat yourself on the back.
- Reframe threats into challenges.
- Learn to accept compliments
- Plan to feel good. Affirm it until it becomes the truth.

WORKING ON:

_____

_____

_____

_____

_____

_____

_____

_____

_____

18 HOW TO DO AFFIRMATIONS

If you change mentally, your body will follow physically. If you care about that mental image of what you want for yourself enough, you will work at the mental part as hard, if not harder, than you work for it physically. You may think you are working hard for changes now, but everything will really work better and happen faster if you do it through affirmations and learn to do them properly.

"In the jungle you will either think about the bullets being fired at you, or where you are aiming, but not both. I always choose to think about where I am aiming and where I am going. This leads to massive productivity. The deep training of your mind to do this instinctively is the single most valuable thing you can have on this earth." —Bob Samara, US Army K-9 Corps, Vietnam Point Man

Do you believe in the law of attraction? Do you believe that thoughts are energy and that what you think about you bring about? Everything you have and are right now *is* a result of your thoughts, beliefs, and what you've brought about. You can bring the scale to the weight you desire because you think you can, believe you can, and are doing things to make it happen. You truly believe that, don't you? Affirmations are goals in motion with thoughts and belief and the power of affirmative energy. Likewise, prayers are simply goals with wings on them. Whether you label it *prayer* or pure *affirmations*, when you ask and believe, you are given abundantly.

How do we know? Lee went from being unable to lose more than a pound a month on any diet for four years to losing 90 pounds in less than eight months. She did affirmations and went from $1.67 and being totally broke to having a chain of weight loss clinics and being successful beyond belief. When she coauthored her first book, we all visualized and did affirmations, and it hit number twenty-one on Amazon's bestseller list. Do you think it just happened? We planned for it to happen: affirmed it, visualized it, prayed about it, and claimed it.

Lee's mentor once told her, "You will do your affirmations to the extent you care about your future." Lee says, "Of course, he had to say it for *years* before I actually got it and really heard it. Now it rings in my head almost daily: 'You will do your affirmations to the extent you care about your future!' "

If you ever get the opportunity to go to one of Bob Samara's IMAGE seminars, "Psychology for Wellness," please go so that you can learn from the master how to do them. (IMAGE stands for intuition, motivation, awareness, genius, and energy.) He was teaching "The Secret" before we knew there *was* a secret. His method of teaching will open a new dimension for you in every area of your life that just studying the Law of Attraction cannot.

The following instructions and affirmations are things we learned from Samara. To list them here does not adequately do you justice. I have yet to meet anyone that would follow the instructions properly or who could write their own affirmations without innocently injecting the wrong information in their brain. DO NOT TRY TO MAKE UP YOUR OWN OR VARY FROM THESE without the help of Bob Samara or Bob Proctor or someone of that caliber helping you. It is too important to your success and to how your are reprogramming your brain.

Instructions for Weight Loss Affirmations
1) It is critical that you follow these exactly as written and not modified to suit you.
2) They must be done twice a day without fail at these specific times: before you get out of bed in the morning and before you go to sleep but are in bed.

3) Must be done in first-person, present tense only.
4) Must be done in the positive, never negative.
5) They should be reviewed by someone experienced in the law of attraction or affirmations before you proceed.
6) Put them on index cards or spiral bound three-by-five index cards so that you can change them as you meet you goals, and add others besides weight loss affirmations.

Weight Loss Affirmations
- I have abundant energy and vitality.
- I choose to make healthy positive choices for myself.
- I eat like the thin person I am.
- I have high self-esteem, and I love me!
- I am at the right place, doing the right thing at the right time, all the time.
- I have the ability to handle every situation.
- I am building a storehouse of energy.
- I do all I can everyday to make a loving environment for all around me.
- Everybody around me knows how much I love them.
- I love and care for my body.
- I always eat the right portions.
- I am always prepared for my nutritional plan for the day and week.
- I love the compliments I get at _____ pounds (goal weight), and it is easy to maintain this healthy weight.
- Exercise is a regular part of my life and I always find things I enjoy to do.
- I am cool, calm, and collected at all times.
- I know when to say "no" to people and put myself first.
- I am truly grateful for everything in my life and live a life of gratitude.
- Everybody around me knows how much I appreciate them.
- Everything turns out exquisitely better than I could have ever planned.

For affirmations to work, I mean *really* work, you have to treat them as if everything depends on it, because it does! *Everything* depends on how well and how often you do your affirmations. And you *must* do them daily for them to work. Remember the car analogy from the introduction? Your body is the only one you are going to get. When you do affirmations, you are spit-shining your aura! You will have a new attitude to motivate you. You are going to glow! Your vehicle will be noticed! Yes!

TIP: Affirmations done in conjunction with goal setting is very powerful. The best system we have found for that is a system that will help you track and visualize all your goals on your computer or mobile phone: http://www.goalsontrack.com.

Get off the merry-go-round of diet after diet and stick to one nutritional plan to lose your weight. The next time you diet, make a real commitment to stick to whatever plan you choose, and not just to the diet phase—you have to commit to the maintenance phase and beyond. Don't just "do a diet" temporarily—make it a nutritional change *for life*. Once you lose the weight, do the maintenance plan continuing to use the tips you have found in this book, and commit to be fit with a nutrition and exercise plan for the rest of your long and healthy life. No more emotional triggers, because you will fix them and get the help you need. You will do the work on yourself while you work on your weight. No excuses. You are too important. You will upgrade your mental software by faithfully doing affirmations every morning and every night. Your commitment is a lifestyle of continually embracing healthy choices in eating, exercising, and everything you do. And then, everything will turn out exquisitely better than you plan it!

MY AFFIRMATIONS:

_____

_____

_____

_____

_____

Answers to Quiz from Chapter 1

Protein	Carbohydrates	Fats
meat	bread	cheese
eggs	cucumbers	butter
beef	berries	creamer
fish	grapefruit	peanut butter
chicken	broccoli	
milk	toast	
yogurt	green beans	
cheese	squash	

NOTES:_____

_____

_____

_____

_____

_____

_____

_____

_____

_____

_____

Foods suitable on a low-fodmap diet

fruit	vegetables	grain foods	milk products	other
fruit	**vegetables**	**cereals**	**milk**	**sweeteners**
banana, blueberry, boysenberry, cantaloupe, cranberry, durian, grape, grapefruit, honeydew melon, kiwifruit, lemon, lime, mandarin, orange, passionfruit, pawpaw, raspberry, rhubarb, rockmelon, star anise, strawberry, tangelo	alfalfa, artichoke, bamboo shoots, bean shoots, bok choy, carrot, celery, choko, choy sum, endive, ginger, green beans, lettuce, olives, parsnip, potato, pumpkin, red capsicum (bell pepper), silver beet, spinach, summer squash (yellow), swede, sweet potato, taro, tomato, turnip, yam, zucchini	gluten-free bread or cereal products	lactose-free milk, oat milk*, rice milk, soy milk*	sugar* (sucrose), glucose, artificial sweeteners not ending in '-ol'
		bread	*check for additives	**honey substitutes**
		100% spelt bread		golden syrup*, maple syrup*, molasses, treacle
		rice	**cheeses**	
Note: if fruit is dried, eat in small quantities		**oats**	hard cheeses, and brie and camembert	*small quantities
	herbs	**polenta**	**yoghurt**	
	basil, chili, coriander, ginger, lemongrass, marjoram, mint, oregano, parsley, rosemary, thyme	**other**	lactose-free varieties	
		arrowroot, millet, psyllium, quinoa, sorgum, tapioca	**ice-cream substitutes**	
			gelati, sorbet	
			butter substitutes	
			olive oil	

Eliminate foods containing fodmaps

excess fructose	lactose	fructans	galactans	polyols
fruit	**milk**	**vegetables**	**legumes**	**fruit**
apple, mango, nashi, pear, tinned fruit in natural juice, watermelon	milk from cows, goats or sheep, custard, ice cream, yoghurt	asparagus, beetroot, broccoli, brussels sprouts, cabbage, eggplant, fennel, garlic, leek, okra, onion (all), shallots, spring onion	baked beans, chickpeas, kidney beans, lentils	apple, apricot, avocado, blackberry, cherry, lychee, nashi, nectarine, peach, pear, plum, prune, watermelon
sweeteners	**cheeses**			**vegetables**
fructose, high fructose corn syrup	soft unripened cheeses eg. cottage, cream, mascarpone, ricotta	**cereals**		cauliflower, green capsicum (bell pepper), mushroom, sweet corn
large total fructose dose		wheat and rye, in large amounts eg. bread, crackers, cookies, couscous, pasta		**sweeteners**
concentrated fruit sources, large serves of fruit, dried fruit, fruit juice		**fruit**		sorbitol (420), mannitol (421), isomalt (953), maltitol (965), xylitol (967)
honey		custard apple, persimmon, watermelon		
corn syrup, fruisana		**miscellaneous**		
		chicory, dandelion, inulin		

ABOUT THE AUTHORS

Lee McCaskill is the founder and CEO of Before and After Weight Loss Clinics and the nationwide diet program, The Belly Buster Diet, and its parent company, Diet Resources International. She majored in Microbiology at Clemson University minored in Food Science. Lee is a Master Certified Weight Loss and Wellness Coach, as well as a microbiologist and herbologist who formulates many of the companies' unique products, including Tropical Spa Body Wraps. She is the author of three cookbooks and a co-author of the bestselling book, *Wake Up...Live the Life You Love: Living in Clarity*.

Michael Vernon is a Bachelor of Science graduate of The Ohio State University, and a former US Navy Pilot. He is a behavioral modification coach for Before and After Weight Loss Clinics and is the Vice President of Belly Buster Diet, Inc. He is also the chairman of a motion picture corporation, Master Poker Face Productions, Inc, and the president of Operation: America Loves You (http://www.opsaly.org/), a 501-c-3 non-profit organization that works to boost the morale of American servicemen and women. Michael is the author of book and screenplay *The Hot Dog Harry Story*.

Facebook: http://www.facebook.com/bellybuster
Twitter: @bellybuster
http://www.bestdietsource.com/
http://www.tropicalspawraps.com/

For more information on clinics or products or to order more books, call (772) 429-1110 or 1-888-657-5402.

www.ingramcontent.com/pod-product-compliance
Lightning Source LLC
Chambersburg PA
CBHW061721020426
42331CB00006B/1030

9780986400520